Voices of Scleroderma
Volume 3

Voices of Scleroderma
Volume 3

Editors
Judith Thompson Devlin & Shelley L. Ensz
for the
International Scleroderma Network

ISN Press

Voices of Scleroderma Volume 3, First Edition

Editors Judith Thompson Devlin and Shelley L. Ensz
Senior Editors Sonya Detwiler, Maia Dock, Lynda Seminara
Production Shelley Ensz
Cover Art Ione Bridgman
Cover Art Assistant Sherrill Knaggs
Distribution Christine Patane

Published by ISN Press7455 France Avenue South, #266, Edina, MN 55435.

Printed and bound in the United States of America.

Disclaimer: We do not endorse or recommend any treatment for scleroderma or related illnesses. Please consult your doctor or scleroderma expert for treatment advice.

Sources: All personal stories in this book were originally published on the ww.sclero.org website and are reprinted here with written permission of the authors. Pen names have been used when requested and in many instances, author names are different between the website and book stories. All stories have been edited for clarity and content for this book.

Library of Congress Control Number: 2005909912
Publisher: BookSurge, LLC
North Charleston, South Carolina

ISBN: 0-9724623-2-5

Dedication

Lives of great men all remind us
We can make our lives sublime,
And, departing, leave behind us
Footprints on the sands of time.

Footprints, that perhaps another,
Sailing o'er life's solemn main,
A forlorn and shipwrecked brother,
Seeing, shall take heart again.

Let us then be up and doing,
With a heart for any fate;
Still achieving, still pursuing,
Learn to labor and to wait.

— Henry Wadsworth Longfellow
From "A Psalm of Life"

To all the great people herein who are still achieving
and still pursuing by letting their voice be heard
in the worldwide labor to conquer scleroderma,
"the disease that turns people to stone."

Table of Contents

Part 2: Juvenile and Localized Scleroderma

Chapter 5: Juvenile Scleroderma

Juvenile Scleroderma by Fernanda Falcini, M.D.

Chapter 6: Localized Scleroderma (Linear and Morphea)

Linear

Morphea

Part 4: International

◆❖◆

Acknowledgments

by Judith Thompson Devlin and Shelley L. Ensz

Judith Thompson Devlin is Chair of the Archivist Committee for the International Scleroderma Network (ISN). Shelley Ensz is Founder and President of the International Scleroderma Network, the ISN's Scleroderma from A to Z Web site at www.sclero.org, and the Scleroderma Webmaster's Association.

This book features over one hundred stories and was created by over one hundred and fifty global volunteers who have worked together via the Internet, cutting across all the barriers of language and politics to share information and support with each other.

All the proceeds of this book series will benefit the nonprofit patient organization, the International Scleroderma Network (ISN).

Certainly, the first credit for this book goes to everyone who has shared their story on ISN's *Scleroderma from A to Z* website where these stories were first posted and where the inspiration for this book was born. These stories are the heart, the soul, and the lifeblood of the website where we all first met and the international nonprofit that we became.

Many thanks go to Arnold Slotkin, a dear friend who calmly insisted that forming the ISN nonprofit would be a fitting outgrowth of the website, despite Shelley's many objections. He gracefully weathered many emails spouting, "Arnold, this is all your fault!" But, of course, it is really to his everlasting credit.

Shelley also extends hearty thanks to Judith, for this book and series would not have existed without her enthusiastic urging and leadership. Judith generously volunteered to archive this series the day after the ISN was publicly launched on January 21, 2002.

ISN board members who were more heavily involved with the launching of this book series include Gene Ensz and Nolan LaTourelle. Linda K. Hopkins of Intelliware International Law Firm, who is Chair of the ISN Legal Advisory Council, provided invaluable advice for this series.

Ione Bridgman, who is an ISN Artist, painted our beautiful cover design to illustrate this book's theme of challenge, with the inspiring mountain scene. Sherrill Knaggs created the digital art from Ione's painting.

Senior editors for this book were Sonya Detwiler, Maia Dock and Lynda Seminara. We are enormously grateful for their wisdom, skill and persistence in polishing this manuscript.

Christine Patane, who is ISN Membership and Donation Coordinator, did the final verification of mailing addresses for this book series and prepared the shipping labels for the first edition books which were signed and sent by Judith Thompson Devlin.

The ISN Medical Advisory Board is led by Dr. James Seibold, who has written the Introduction to this volume. He is Professor of Internal Medicine and Director of the University of Michigan Scleroderma Program in Ann Arbor, Michigan. Author of more than three hundred scientific publications, he is considered a world thought leader in scleroderma, Raynaud's phenomenon, and interventional research in the rheumatologic diseases.

Professional contributors to this volume also nclude Dr. Marco Matucci-Cerinic, Dr. Irene Miniati, Dr. Fernanda Falcini, Dr. László Czirják, Dr. Tafazzul e-Haque Mahmud, Francisco J. Castellanos, and Carol Langenfeld.

Dr. Marco Matucci-Cerinic is Professor of Rheumatology and Medicine and Director of Division of Medicine and Rheumatology, at the University of Florence, Italy. He is also Chairman of the EULAR Scleroderma Trial and Research group (EUSTAR), Vice President of the Scleroderma Clinical Trials Consortium (SCTC), and serves on the ISN Medical Advisory Board. He and Dr. Miniati are our featured experts for this volume, with the lead article in *Chapter 1*, which is an overview of systemic scleroderma.

Dr. Irene Miniati is a rheumatologist in the Division of Medicine & Rheumatology at the University of Florence, Italy, whose principal field of interest is autologous stem cell transplantation in scleroderma.

Dr. Fernanda Falcini is a pediatric rheumatologist in the Department of Pediatrics, University of Florence, Italy. Her introduction to juvenile scleroderma is graced with child-friendly illustrations by Sherrill Knaggs.

Professor László Czirják is head of the Department of Immunology and Rheumatology at the Hungarian Brothers of St. John of God and University of Pécs, Irgalmasok, Hungary. He also serves on the Board of Counsellors for EULAR Scleroderma Trials and Research (EUSTAR) organization. His review of scleroderma-like disorders explores the broad range of similar ailments, as well as their underlying causes.

Dr. Tafazzul e-Haque Mahmud is Assistant Professor and in charge of the Rheumatology Unit at Shaikh Zayed Federal Postgraduate Medical Institute, a teaching hospital in Lahore, Pakistan. He serves on the ISN Medical Advisory Board. Like many of our scleroderma experts, the tragic death of a scleroderma patient inspired his dedication to rheumatology, so he wrote the introduction to our chapter of Stories in Remembrance.

Francisco J. Castellanos is Founder and President of the Asociación Colombiana de Esclerodermia, which is an affiliate of the International Scleroderma Network. His article is the introduction to the Spanish chapter.

Carol Langenfeld, MSEd, PC, NCC, is a professional counselor who has lived with scleroderma since 1977 and also has the experience of being a caregiver for her husband Doug during his long-time illness. They co-authored a book sharing the lessons they learned called *Living Better: Every Patient's Guide to Living with Illness*. Carol is a National Certified Counselor and a Licensed Professional Counselor in the State of Ohio.

All stories in this book are printed in their original language and many of them have also been translated into English. Translators for stories that appear in this book include Kevin Howell, Edwin Lamoli-Torres, and Ans Mens. Additionally, dozens of other translators are involved in the preparation and maintenance of our multilingual website.

Kevin Howell is a Clinical Scientist for Professor Carol Black at the Royal Free Hospital in London. His scientific article on measuring microcirculation was in Voices of Scleroderma Volume 2, and in this volume he translated Italian stories.

Edwin Lamoli-Torres is a retired professor from the University of Puerto Rico at Mayaguez. Edwin received his Master's Degree in ESL from Teacher's College, Columbia University in New York City. He translated a Spanish patient story for this volume.

Ans Mens is a former nurse in the Netherlands, who has been an ISN Translator for many years, having founded *Sclerodermie von A tot Z*, which is the Dutch version of our site.

This book was published with funding from the Audrey Love Charitable Foundation, for which we are very grateful.

Please keep in mind that scleroderma affects everyone differently. There is no predictable course for any form of the disease. Nothing in this book is intended as personal medical advice, so please consult your doctor before making any changes to lifestyle or treatments. We do our best to keep the most current information on treatments and clinical trials available on our website.

With so many people involved in this book's production, the only thing for certain is that there are countless people who have played a vital role in its success who are not mentioned here. Many of them are profiled on our website as ISN representatives or supporters. Some of our volunteers prefer to work anonymously or behind the scenes. Their names deserve to be here also, and they are woven throughout this book in spirit.

We hope it will suffice to say that if you have ever helped the cause of scleroderma in any way, anywhere in the world, you have done a great and grand deed, and we are all very thankful for your footprints in the sand.

Introduction
by James R. Seibold, M.D.

Dr. Seibold is Chair of the ISN Medical Advisory Board. He is Professor of Internal Medicine and Director of the University of Michigan Scleroderma Program in Ann Arbor, Michigan, USA.

We welcome you to *Voices of Scleroderma*, a major contribution from the International Scleroderma Network (ISN).

Scleroderma occurs in only around thirty people per million per year. Therefore, since it is so uncommon, patients have great difficulty finding access to expert care or even another similarly afflicted patient with whom they can share their experience.

Access to high quality reliable modern information is crucial to patient well-being and outcomes. The realization that "you ARE NOT alone" has therapeutic value in its own right.

I'm privileged to Chair the ISN Medical Advisory, and also serve as President of the Scleroderma Clinical Trials Consortium (SCTC). The SCTC is an international charitable organization of academic centers dedicated to elevating the pace and quality of scleroderma research. The SCTC works closely with the ISN in the education of both patients and caregivers.

The ISN is active on a wide variety of fronts, most notably in the shared goal of providing up to date and accurate information to the scleroderma community on a worldwide basis. Over the past eight years, I have watched the amazing development of the Web site that Shelley Ensz created at www.sclero.org. I have seen it evolve from her personal site of one page to become the ISN site, now encompassing over twelve hundred pages in twenty-two languages. Over 1.2 million visits were made to the ISN Web site this year alone. The ISN is the major worldwide source of information about scleroderma.

The ISN site has brought together both the medical and patient communities from throughout the world. According to all the major ranking services of Internet traffic, it is in the top 225,000 of all Web sites, far ahead of all other scleroderma-related sites.

In my view, the primary reason for this stellar success is the high quality of site content, as well as the multilingual, international reach, which is also an important driving force. Remarkably, the ISN has a small team of committed, dedicated volunteers who have seized the amazing capabilities of the Internet to provide exceptional, worldwide service and assistance to patients with scleroderma.

More notably, from this enterprising site, the ISN has in turn developed into a thriving nonprofit organization. It is really a classic example of reversing the order of development. Rather than an established organization simply developing a Web site, a remarkably effective Web site developed into a full-service charitable organization.

The ISN expands upon its cyberspace outreach by publishing *Voices of Scleroderma*. Every volume in this book series features articles from esteemed scleroderma researchers as well as over one hundred patient and caregiver stories, from sixteen countries, and in five languages.

The ISN enjoys a well-deserved reputation for top-notch medical and support information and services from both the patient and medical organizations throughout the world. Today, over five dozen dedicated volunteers, including many doctors and translators, operate the ISN.

Our ISN Medical Advisory Board includes illustrious experts in this field, such as Dr. Luis Catoggio of Buenos Aires, Argentina; Dr. Marco Matucci-Cerinic of Florence, Italy; Dr. C. Stephen Foster of Boston, Massachusetts; Dr. Frank van den Hoogen of The Netherlands; Dr. Hsiao-Yi Lin of Taiwan; Dr. Tafazzul e-Haque Mahmud of Lahore, Pakistan; Dr. Janet Pope of London, Ontario; and Dr. Shinichi Sato of Kanazawa, Japan.

Dozens of other renowned leaders in their field also generously lend their expertise to the ISN, primarily as contributing authors, medical editors, scientific advisors, and translators.

All of our ISN volunteers met and work only through the Internet. Their efforts have made quality medical and support information on this rare disease available worldwide.

I hope you find this book of value, and that you also consider offering support to the ISN. It is only with a partnership of patients and scientists in a concerted worldwide effort that we will solve the riddle of scleroderma.

◆❖◆

PART 1

Systemic Scleroderma

CHAPTER 1

Systemic Scleroderma
Medical Information

*Systemic sclerosis patients, and particularly those with
early aggressive disease, should be treated
in specialized scleroderma centers.*

—Professor Marco Matucci-Cerinic

Systemic Sclerosis
by Marco Matucci-Cerinic, M.D. and Irene Miniati, M.D.

Dr. Marco Matucci-Cerinic is Professor of Rheumatology and Medicine and Director of Division of Medicine & Rheumatology, University of Florence, Italy. He is also Chairman of the EULAR Scleroderma Trial and Research group (EU-STAR), Vice President of the Scleroderma Clinical Trials Consortium (SCTC), and serves on the ISN Medical Advisory Board.

Dr. Irene Miniati is a rheumatologist in the Division of Medicine & Rheumatology at the University of Florence, Italy, whose principal field of interest is autologous stem cell transplantation in scleroderma.

What Is Systemic Sclerosis?

Systemic sclerosis (SSc) is a chronic inflammatory disease that affects the connective tissue and is characterized by excessive fibrosis of the skin and internal organs.

The disease is commonly called "scleroderma" because the most visible aspect is "hard skin." The progressive skin thickening, caused by sclerosis of the derma, typically appears in the face and hands, where joint contractures can be observed.

However, scleroderma is a systemic disease and because of its potential aggressiveness, it was termed *"the most terrible of human ills"* by Sir William Osler.[1] Besides the significant aesthetic changes of the face and extremities, organ involvement may lead to a functional reduction, sometimes progressing to end-stage failure.

The cause that triggers this disease is still unknown. Microcirculation, the immune system, and connective tissue are involved in the tissue damage evolving to the final step, fibrosis. The mechanisms that connect these systems and result in the disease are still not clear.

Two subsets of systemic sclerosis have been observed: "limited cutaneous" and "diffuse cutaneous." The former is characterized by skin involvement limited to the face and extremities, with late internal organ involvement. The latter has more rapid evolution, with early internal organ involvement that can lead to death in just a few years.

Prevalence of the Disease

Although SSc is a relatively uncommon disease, rough estimates based on United States data indicate that every year 20 people per million are diagnosed with SSc. It is believed that approximately 240 people per million now suffer from this disease. However, there is not sufficient epidemiological information to precisely quantify the number of people affected.

More women than men are afflicted with SSc. Some studies have suggested that SSc is induced by exposure to certain environmental elements such as cleaning products, solvents, silica dust, and working with vibratory tools such as chain saws and drills.

Onset of the Disease

The first symptom of systemic sclerosis (SSc) is Raynaud's phenomenon (RP) of the fingers, toes, ears, and nose. Raynaud's is characterized by episodic vasospastic attacks that cause the blood vessels in the fingers and toes to constrict or narrow. The blood supply to the extremities is greatly decreased.

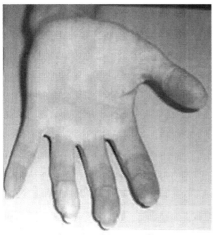

Attack of Raynaud's with whiteness (pallor) of 4th finger, and blueness (cyanosis) of the others.
J. Devlin, ISN Photo Repository

Raynaud's presents with three changes in skin color. Pallor (in response to spasm of the arterioles and the resulting collapse of digital arteries) is followed by cyanosis (due to ischemia) and finally, as the arterioles dilate and blood returns to the digits, rubor occurs. The duration of an attack varies from less than one minute to several hours. As the attack ends, throbbing and tingling may occur in the fingers and toes.

Suffering from Raynaud's does not mean that one is necessarily affected by systemic sclerosis. In fact, most people with Raynaud's have no underlying disease or associated medical problem (this is the "primary" form of Raynaud's). Women are affected more often than men, especially those between 15 and 40 years of age.

When an underlying disease or condition causes Raynaud's it is referred to as "secondary" RP. Connective tissue diseases, such as scleroderma, are the most common cause of secondary RP.

Nail-fold capillaroscopy (study of capillaries under a microscope) can help the physician distinguish between primary and secondary RP. During this test, a drop of oil is placed on the patient's nail folds (the skin at the base of the fingernail) and examined under a microscope for abnormalities of the tiny blood vessels (capillaries). If nail-fold video-capillaroscopy (NVC) shows a variety of morphological and quantitative changes, the patient may have a connective tissue disease.

Ulcers may arise as a complication of RP and chronic ischemia, resulting from a combination of functional and structural changes of the small vessels. Ulcers occur most frequently on the fingertips or over the interphalangeal joints and generally are painful. Because of the peripheral ischemia, the regenerative/reparative capacities of tissues are reduced. Thus, ulcers heal slowly and become portals for infections.

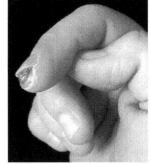

Digital Ulcer. on Fingertip.
ISN Photo Repository.

Ulcers may evolve to gangrene and, as they deepen into the tissues, bone involvement can occur, which may result in osteomyelitis. In the worst cases, digital amputation may be needed.

Primary Clinical Features

The disease has various clinical characteristics because it involves the skin as well as the internal organs. At onset, some patients present with few changes and without significant hematologic modifications (such as antibodies), making the diagnosis difficult to establish even for scleroderma experts. This may explain why the diagnosis is usually made once the disease has fully developed. However, early diagnosis is essential for starting appropriate treatment aimed at blocking disease evolution.

Below is an in-depth description of the various types of internal organ involvement observed in SSc.

Gastrointestinal Tract Involvement

Fibrosis can involve the entire gastrointestinal (GI) tract, making the muscle wall of these organs atrophic. Damage to the gut's nervous system may cause dysmotility.

Upper Tract

Esophageal disease is characterized by poor functioning of the muscle of the lower part of the esophagus. This causes a reduction of the rhythmic motion that propels food toward the stomach (called peristalsis) and of the continence of the sphinteric junction between the esophagus and stomach (called lower esophageal sphincter [LES]). This is a thick circular ring of smooth muscle at the bottom of the esophagus that relaxes before the esophagus contracts, and allows food to pass through to the stomach.

After a meal, it usually remains closed to prevent acid and food particles from refluxing into the esophagus. The reduced ability of the esophagus to move food down into the stomach is caused by an abnormality of peristaltic movements. This often manifests as difficulty or pain during swallowing (called dysphagia).

In addition, the defect of continence of the LES and an abnormally wide esophagus can lead to reflux episodes that irritate the tissue of the lower part of esophagus, causing heartburn, pyrosis, and regurgitation.

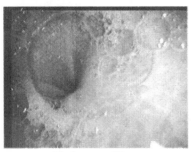

Endoscopy View
Lower Third of the Esophagus
E. Ensz, ISN Photo Repository

Other less common symptoms are sore throat, laryngitis, inflammation of the gums, erosion of tooth enamel, chronic irritation in the throat, and hoarseness in the morning.

Sometimes there are no symptoms, and the presence of gastroesophageal reflux is revealed through other complications. In a small subset of patients, a complication known as Barrett's esophagus has been identified. This is a potentially precancerous condition in which the mucosa of the esophagus is transformed in an abnormal lining, called "specialized intestinal metaplasia." Patients with such symptoms should be monitored closely with endoscopy in order to start prompt therapy and prevent complications.

Esophageal motility is usually tested by manometry. This test is performed by placing a thin catheter (with several pressure sensors) into the nostril and then positioning it in the stomach. Water (5 mL) is given every 30 seconds to facilitate evaluation of the amplitude (strength), duration (time), velocity (speed), and presence or absence of peristaltic contractions (wave-like movement that propels contents forward) and to determine whether the measurements are within normal range.

To evaluate tissue damage, upper endoscopy is recommended. For this procedure, patients swallow a thin, flexible, lighted tube called an endoscope, which transmits an image of the inside of the esophagus, stomach, and duodenum. This allows the physician to carefully examine the lining of these organs. The scope also blows air into the stomach, expanding the folds and permitting careful examination of the stomach. If Barrett's esophagus is detected, routine endoscopic screening is advised.

For people with symptoms of gastroesophageal reflux, a pH-monitoring test can be performed. A tiny tube is placed into the esophagus and remains there for 24 hours. While the patient goes about normal activities, the test measures when and how much acid comes up into the esophagus.

Treatment of esophageal disease in scleroderma is based, first of all, on modifications in lifestyle. Gravity plays an important role in controlling reflux. To minimize the possibility of heartburn, it is recommended that an upright posture be maintained until a meal is digested.

"Gravity plays an important role in controlling reflux."

If heartburn occurs regularly at night, it might be helpful to raise the head of the bed or insert a triangular wedge at this location to ensure that the esophagus remains above the stomach.

Exertion after a meal should be avoided because it contracts the abdominal muscles and forces food through a weakened sphincter. Small and frequent meals are recommended, as is eating early in the evening so that digestion is completed by bedtime.

Certain foods compromise the sphincter's ability to prevent reflux and are best avoided by patients with reflux. The most problematic are fats, onions, and chocolate. Alcohol often provokes heartburn by compromising the LES, irritating the esophagus, and stimulating stomach acid production.

Popular beverages such as coffee (including decaffeinated), tea, cola, tomato juice, and lemon juice may aggravate symptoms by irritating the esophagus or stimulating the production of stomach acid. Being overweight can promote reflux because excessive abdominal fat puts pressure on the stomach.

The medications prescribed to treat esophagus dysmotility and reflux are promotility agents, H2 blockers, and proton pump inhibitors. Promotility agents help strengthen the sphincter and empty the stomach. H2 blockers reduce the amount of acid produced in the stomach, and proton pump inhibitors limit secretion of acid in the stomach. Because these agents work in different ways, combination therapy employing two or more of these drugs may be especially helpful in controlling symptoms.

The abnormality of the gut's nervous system present in SSc also can involve the stomach's electrical rhythm, with the motility becoming weakened, spastic, or failing completely. In the most severe forms, nausea, vomiting, abdominal pain, and severe constipation are unrelenting.

Gastroparesis, or small bowel dysmotility, is at the extreme end of the symptom spectrum. Gastroparesis is a severe neuromuscular disorder of the stomach that results in a partially or completely paralyzed stomach. Patients suffer from a spectrum of symptoms known as "dyspepsia." The range of symptoms includes nausea, vomiting, belching, stomach acid washing into the mouth (reflux), sensation of fullness after a few bites of food (early satiety), abdominal pain, abdominal bloating, change in bowel habits, and weight loss. Thus, gastroparesis can significantly impact quality of life.

Gastric emptying time (GET) is the diagnostic test used for gastroparesis. The entire upper tract, including the stomach antrum, pylorus, and the duodenum, may all play a role in delayed emptying of the stomach. Individuals may have varying degrees of dysfunction in these GI regions, resulting in delayed stomach emptying. Prokinetic drugs are indicated to promote emptying of the stomach and gut, and to enhance the contractions and coordination of the gut.

Lower Tract

The small bowel can become dilated and often atonic, losing its propulsive function. Under these conditions, bacteria that normally live

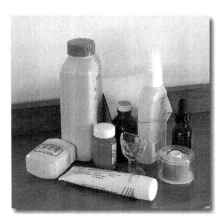

in the small bowel grow enormously, damaging the mucosa that absorbs food. This leads to malabsorption, with significant loss of absorption of fundamental substances.

Symbiotic colonic bacteria normally assist digestion. The upper GI tract was once believed to be sterile, but normal colonization of the duodenum, jejunum, and ileum is now recognized.

Bacterial overgrowth syndrome (BOS) occurs when the normally low colonization of bacteria in the upper GI tract increases significantly. Fat, protein, carbohydrate, and vitamin malabsorption result from poor enterocyte function and from bacterial transformation of nutrients into nonabsorbable and toxic metabolites, all of which contribute to damage in the intestinal mucosa.

Malabsorption and enterocyte dysfunction further degrade the health of the gut by reducing local and systemic nutrition delivery. When bacterial overgrowth is caused by slow transit through the small bowel, broad-spectrum antibiotics are indicated for a few days per month, and patients should reduce or avoid fats and fiber in their diet in an effort to reduce abdominal symptoms such as constipation and distension.

Breath tests using byproducts of bacterial metabolism to identify malabsorbed substances are useful in determining the diagnosis. The most sensitive and specific is the xylose breath test, which is based on the fact that overgrowth of gram-negative bacteria in the small bowel, which occurs during dysmotility disorders, leads to metabolization of xylose and results in the release of radioactive carbon dioxide. One gram of D-xylose tagged with carbon 14 (as a liquid) is administered after an overnight fast. Then the radioactive carbon dioxide is inhaled and measured at 30, 60, 90, and 120 minutes. An abnormally high carbon dioxide concentration is usually de-tected within 30 to 60 minutes.

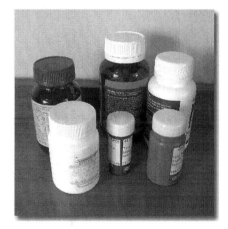

In the most severe cases, bowel dilatation may result in a condition known as intestinal pseudo-obstruc-tion. In such cases, patients should avoid oral feeding and require use of continuous nasogastric suction. When malnutrition is evident, total parenteral nutrition (using a central venous catheter) is indicated.

The intestinal nervous system also can be involved; contractions that normally move food into the bowel are reduced in intensity and frequency. Thus, the bowel remains atonic and nonpropulsive, causing fermentation and bacterial overgrowth. In early phases, treatment with octreotide can stimulate small bowel function, helping to reduce bacterial overgrowth.

The colon can become atonic and dilated, developing wide-mouthed diverticulae. This can sometimes cause diverticulitis owing to bacterial proliferation and, although rare, rupture can occur.

In some patients, fecal (bowel) incontinence develops from weaken-ing of the anal sphincter. Electrical devices may be used to stimulate the anal sphincter. In such cases, anorectal manometry is indicated. With this procedure, a thin catheter is placed in the anorectal sphincter to evaluate peristaltic contractions. This same technique is usually performed for upper tract dysmotility.

Lung Involvement

The primary function of the respiratory system is to supply the blood with oxygen to be delivered throughout the body. The exchange of oxygen between the air we breath and our blood takes place in the alveoli, which are tiny air sacs that develop from the bronchiolar arms at the end of the respiratory tract. Normally a small amount of connective tissue separates alveoli from capillaries that contain red blood cells and act as oxygen carriers.

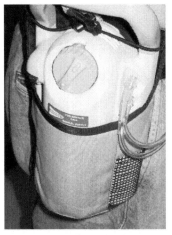

In systemic scleroderma (SSc), the amount of this connective tissue is increased, scarring the tissue and thickening their walls. The extent of scarring and fibrosis varies from mild to extensive.

Cough and a sensation of breathlessness on exertion are the earliest symptoms of lung involvement. Depending on the severity of the condition, simple activities such as walking or talking on the telephone may become increasingly difficult, and supplemental oxygen may be required.

Lung involvement may be investigated with pulmonary function tests (PFTs), which are noninvasive and require breathing into a tube via a mouthpiece. Some patients may not be able to accommodate a standard mouthpiece because of oral opening reduction. In such instances, an adapter or a pediatric mouthpiece may be used.

Forced vital capacity (FVC), which measures the total amount of air capable of being blown forcefully, and the diffusion capacity for carbon monoxide (DLCO), a measure of how well oxygen diffuses into blood, are the most important functional measures. PFTs should be repeated at least twice a year in order to accurately evaluate the progression of lung involvement, especially if dyspnea (shortness of breath) worsens.

The overall efficiency of respiration can be estimated by measuring the amount of oxygen saturation in the blood. This can be done by directly measuring oxygen in a sample of arterial blood gases (ABG), or it can be estimated by using a noninvasive instrument known as an oximeter, which fits on the finger, earlobe, or forehead.

A routine chest X ray may demonstrate fibrosis, but it is not very sensitive for detecting early or mild disease. For this reason, a high-resolution computed tomographic (HRCT) scan is required. This noninvasive investigation provides images of multiple slices through the lung, from top (apex) to bottom (base), and can even detect lung involvement in early phases when no symptoms are present.

Bronchoscopy with broncho-alveolar lavage (BAL) is an invasive test that also may provide information about the inflammatory status of the affected areas of the lung detected during HRCT. BAL is performed by a bronchologist, on a conscious-but-sedated patient. It consists of washing a sample of cells and secretions from the alveolar and bronchial airspaces by introducing a commercial sterile saline solution via fiberoptic bronchoscope, which has been wedged into a bronchus. The fluid is then immediately withdrawn. The instilled fluid fills the airspaces distal to the tip of bronchoscope, replacing the air. A portion of the instilled volume remains, to be absorbed or coughed up after the procedure. The cells within this fluid are counted, and a high number of cells demonstrates alveolar inflammation.

Treatment of scleroderma lung disease depends on the extent of lung fibrosis, the degree of inflammatory activity (alveolitis), and the degree of respiratory impairment. When alveolar inflammation is detected, immunosuppressive drugs are required. Supplemental oxygen may be required, when exercising or at rest, for patients whose lung fibrosis leads to significant impairment in providing oxygen to the tissues.

Pulmonary arterial hypertension (PAH) is a serious and potentially life-threatening condition that can develop in patients with scleroderma. It occurs when the blood vessels supplying the lungs constrict and then become stiffer and thicker because of the irreversible fibrosis. The increased resistance in pulmonary circulation makes it difficult for blood to flow through to the lung vessels, and thus the heart must pump harder.

Some patients may have both interstitial lung disease and PAH; the first usually develops early in the disease, whereas PAH tends to occur later, often in the second decade of disease.

The precise cause of PAH is unknown, but it is associated with dysregulation of blood flow that results in vasoconstriction, as is observed in Raynaud's phenomenon. Many factors may play a role in this process; one of them is the elevation of the bodily substance endothelin, a potent vasoconstrictor that has been shown to be elevated in the blood of scleroderma patients and in lung tissue affected by scleroderma.

In the earliest stages of PAH, the patient may not have any symptoms. Then shortness of breath may develop (dyspnea), which generally occurs on exertion in the beginning, and later during ordinary activity. Other symptoms such as chest pain, dizziness, and fainting also may occur, but they are nonspecific. Because of its poor outcome, it is critical that PAH be detected in an early phase, so that prompt therapy can be initiated while the condition is still reversible.

It is recommended that color Doppler echocardiography be performed 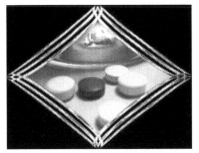 periodically in SSc patients, including those who do not have any symptoms of PAH. This technique can determine the size of the chambers of the heart and how well the heart valves are working. It also estimates pulmonary arterial pressure.

Once PAH is diagnosed, right-heart catheterization can confirm the diagnosis. This procedure entails inserting a thin plastic tube (catheter) into an artery or vein in the arm or leg, which is advanced into the "right heart" or into the coronary arteries. It measures pressure within the heart and the amount of oxygen in the blood. During this procedure, vasodilator drugs can be tested to determine whether they can significantly reduce pulmonary pressure, which may lead to their use as a treatment modality.

The target of therapy is to relax and open blood vessels to facilitate blood flow into the lungs (vasodilation). In some patients, calcium channel blockers (such as nifedifine or diltiazem) are effective. Bosentan, an endothelin receptor antagonist, has been proven to offer several important benefits to patients with PAH, such as reduced dyspnea and improved ability to perform normal daily activities.

Recently a new medication for people with advanced forms of pulmonary arterial hypertension (PAH) was approved by the US Food and Drug Administration. Ventavis®, an inhaled-solution form of iloprost, is indicated for patients classified as having stage III or IV pulmonary hypertension. Iloprost, a prostacyclin analog, is designed to widen abnormally narrowed blood vessels. The drug also is aimed at improving blood circulation and exercise capacity in patients with PAH.

Heart Involvement

Cardiac involvement is common in systemic sclerosis (SSc), and contributes to symptoms such as shortness of breath, fatigue, and palpitations. The heart is often affected subclinically, by a patchy fibrosis involving both the myocardium and the conducting system.

Tachyarrhythmias are excessively rapid and irregular heartbeats. They usually don't cause any symptoms, but they are often fatal, and SSc patients with heart involvement are susceptible to tachyarrhythmias. Thus, a thorough heart-function screening and appropriate follow-up monitoring are mandatory for all SSc patients.

The screening consists of various simple, noninvasive investigations (physical examination, electrocardiogram, chest X ray, Doppler bidimensional echocardiogram) that provide information on the presence of rhythm and conduction disturbances, cardiac morphology and function, and the possible presence of pulmonary arterial hypertension (PAH).

When needed, additional tests may be performed, including long-term ambulatory electrocardiographic recording, assessment of cardiopulmonary performance by the six-minute walking test or cardiopulmonary stress test, cardiac catheterization (mandatory to confirm and better estimate PAH), cardiac magnetic resonance imaging, and nuclear studies of myocardial function and perfusion.

Kidney Involvement

Kidney (renal) involvement in SSc is often clinically silent. It may progress slowly toward renal failure and thus heavily influence prognosis. In some cases, breakdown of the renal system may be abrupt, without any sentinel symptom.

Color Doppler ultrasonography can confirm the early reduction of renal arterial blood flow in patients

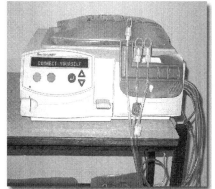

Peritoneal Dialysis Machine

with systemic sclerosis (SSc) who have no clinical sign of renal involvement. Abnormal findings on renal function tests (serum creatinine, creatinine clearance, 24-hour proteinuria) may be observed at a later stage of the disease.

Sudden onset of high blood pressure and kidney failure is known as scleroderma renal crisis (SRC). This usually occurs in patients with diffuse scleroderma, resulting in kidney failure within a few days. Thus, to detect sudden kidney failure promptly, daily at-home monitoring of blood pressure is recommended for systemic sclerosis (SSc) patients, and particularly for those with diffuse scleroderma, even if they do not have high blood pressure or other renal symptoms.

The outcome of scleroderma renal crisis is poor despite aggressive treatment for high blood pressure. SSc patients who develop high blood pressure should immediately receive acetylcholine esterase (ACE) inhibitors to control blood pressure. ACE inhibitors can improve the prognosis, but it is still not known if they can prevent scleroderma renal crisis. Patients with loss of renal function require dialysis.

The Burden of Systemic Sclerosis

The loss of organ function is responsible for the high social and economic impact on national health care systems. Systemic sclerosis (SSc) patients may require continuous assistance at home and various types of medical approaches (rheumatology, pneumology, cardiology, gastroenterology, etc), all of which contribute to the enormous cost of medical care for them. Indeed, the inability to work is another issue that makes the social burden of SSc difficult for health care systems and for patients and their families.

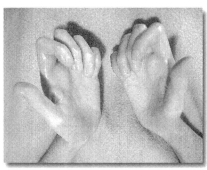

Sclerodactyly:
The final stage of skin fibrosis.
S. Knaggs, ISN Photo Repository

Severe forms of the disease, especially rapidly progressive diffuse systemic sclerosis, is often rapidly fatal due to heart, lung and kidney involvement; about 40%-50% of patients with the worst form of systemic sclerosis (SSc) die within five years.

Fibrosis—the hallmark of systemic sclerosis—is the final step of an inflammatory process, and there is still no treatment proven to reverse fibrosis. That is why early diagnosis of SSc is essential, since adequate treatment of inflammation can prevent the development of fibrosis.

Accurate staging, and a prediction of the damage, are very important for determining appropriate treatment and minimizing disease progression, in turn lessening the chance of irreversible damage and improving overall prognosis.

Unfortunately, many doctors lack the expertise to suspect or detect scleroderma early. Even when they have diagnosed scleroderma, they may not realize the importance of referring patients to specialized scleroderma centers.

Systemic sclerosis patients, and particularly those with early aggressive disease, should be treated in specialized centers familiar with the uniform high standards of sclero-

"Systemic sclerosis patients should be treated in specialized centers."

derma care. These centers can perform biochemistry and instrumental examination necessary for the diagnosis, staging, and follow-up of scleroderma, and provide appropriate care and treatment.

Current Therapies: Limitations and Hope

No proven effective therapy exists to prevent disease progression or to reverse fibrosis. Blinded randomized clinical trials of D-penicillamine and alpha-interferon failed to demonstrate a clinically significant effect. Low-dose oral methotrexate showed beneficial effects on skin thickening, but not on organ dysfunction, in a small placebo-controlled crossover study. Cyclophosphamide has been shown to improve skin thickening, stabilize pulmonary function, and increase survival.

In the past decade, intense immunosuppression followed by autologous stem cells transplantation (HSCT) has emerged as a new therapeutic procedure for patients affected by severe systemic sclerosis (SSc) that has not responded to conventional treatments.

This procedure is intended to eliminate auto-aggressive lymphocytes by a lympho-myeloablative treatment and is followed by stem-cell rescue. A phase I-II trial showed improvement in the skin score, stabilization of lung function and pulmonary pressure, and no occurrence of renal crisis after the treatment. The initial death rate from the procedure was particularly elevated (17%), probably owing to the already advanced organ damage of most participants. The new criteria for patient selection, in terms of both disease stage and organ involvement, have remarkably improved transplant-related survival.

Phase III clinical studies are underway in Europe and the United States. Preliminary results indicate that HSCT can significantly improve skin involvement and stabilize lung function, thus having a positive effect on quality of life.[2]

❖

References

1. William Osler, 1898. "In its more aggravated forms diffuse scleroderma is one of the most terrible of all human ills. Like Tithonus to "wither slowly" and like him to be "beaten down and marred and wasted" until one is literally a mummy, encased in an evershrinking, slowly contracting skin of steel, is a fate not pictured in any tragedy, ancient or modern." Source: Osler, William. On diffuse scleroderma. J Cutan Genitourin Dis. 1898; 16:49 [As cited in Silverman ME, Hurst JW (eds). Clinical Skills for Adult Primary Care. Philadelphia: Lippincott-Raven Publishers; 1996, p. 191].

2. I. Miniati, R. Saccardi, F. Pagliai, L. Lombardini, S. Guidi, C. Nozzoli, A. Bosi, S. Guiducci1, S. Urbani, A. Tyndall, M. Matucci Cerinic. Autologous Stem Cells Transplantation for Severe Diffuse Systemic Sclerosis (SSc): 2 Years of Follow Up. FRI0108, EULAR 2005.

Systemic Scleroderma Symptom Checklist

Please consult your doctor if you have two or more of the following symptoms, which are sometimes due to systemic sclerosis (scleroderma). Systemic scleroderma may disqualify a person for life and/or health insurance in some countries. Sometimes certain lab work or biopsy results may force an unwelcome diagnosis into the medical record.

Circulation
❑ Swelling of hands, feet and/or face
❑ Raynaud's: fingers and/or toes turn white or blue due to cold or stress
❑ Ulcers (sores) on fingertips or toes

Gastrointestinal
❑ Difficulty swallowing
❑ Heartburn (reflux)
❑ Constipation, diarrhea, irritable bowel syndrome

Heart, Lungs, Kidneys
❑ Shortness of breath
❑ Pulmonary (lung) fibrosis
❑ Aspiration pneumonia
❑ Pulmonary hypertension
❑ High blood pressure or kidney (renal) failure
❑ Right-sided heart failure

Muscles & Tendons
❑ Tendonitis, or carpal tunnel syndrome
❑ Muscle aches, weakness, joint pain

Excessive Dryness or Sjögren's Syndrome
❑ Excessive dryness of the mucus membranes (such as eyes, mouth, vagina), which is sometimes called Sjögren's Syndrome

Skin
❑ Tight skin, often on hands or face
❑ Calcinosis (calcium deposits)
❑ Telangiectasia (red dots on the hands or face)
❑ Mouth becomes smaller, lips develop deep grooves, eating and dental care become difficult

Many of these symptoms can occur by themselves or can be due to other things. Symptoms such as heartburn, high blood pressure, constipation, and muscle aches are very common in the general population. More unusual symptoms, such as tight skin and/or pulmonary fibrosis, may be more likely to lead to a scleroderma diagnosis.

◆❖◆

Scleroderma-like Disorders
by László Czirják, M.D.

Professor László Czirják is head of the Department of Immunology and Rheumatology at the Hungarian Brothers of St. John of God and University of Pécs, Irgalmasok, Hungary. He also serves on the Board of Counsellors for EULAR Scleroderma Trials and Research (EUSTAR) organization.

Scleroderma-like disorders usually mimic skin symptoms similar to the classic early skin thickening or late skin atrophy present in "classic" systemic sclerosis (SSc).

A few important signs may indicate that the particular patient does not have SSc, but another related disorder. The distribution/characteristics of skin involvement seem to be "atypical". The lack of the typical scleroderma skin involvement of the digits, and the lack cold sensitivity causing Raynaud's phenomenon may indicate the presence of scleroderma-like disorder. The typical SSc-related internal organ involvements are missing in scleroderma-like diseases.

Skin biopsy is crucial for those with atypical scleroderma-like symptoms.

In patients with systemic sclerosis we usually find scleroderma-specific antinuclear antibodies (anti-centromere, anti-toposiomerase, etc), and the nailfold capillarocopy also shows the typical signs of "scleroderma capillary pattern" in the great majority of cases. Both the lack of specific autoantibodies and the normal capillaroscopy may indicate the presence of a scleroderma-like disease.

In the case history, some patients have an exposure to chemicals or drugs. Skin biopsy is very important in all patients exhibiting atypical scleroderma-like symptoms, therefore this is the crucial investigation that usually provides the final diagnosis. Skin biopsy often shows that the deeper tissues (fascia, muscles) are also abnormal.

There is a very long list of scleroderma-like disorders, and it is difficult to categorize them *(Table 1)*. Mucin deposition is present in an important subgroup of patients. In patients with hypothyroidism, generalized or localized myxedema may mimic systemic sclerosis.

Sclerodemyxedema is characterized by waxy papules with marked skin sclerosis affecting the hands, arms, face and to a lesser extent the trunk and lower extremities. The disease onset is between 30 to 70 years of age. Proximal myopathy, esophageal dysmotility, polyarthritis and central nervous system symptoms may also occur. In patients with scleredema (Buschke), quickly developing, nonpitting indurated edema or stiffness of the skin appears on the neck, shoulder girdle, face, occasionally on the trunk and the proximal part of extremities. The face becomes mask-like. The feet are spared.

Patients with nephrogenic fibrosing dermopathy (NFD) develop large areas of hardened skin with slightly raised plaques, papules, or confluent papules. The symmetrical skin involvement affects the trunk and the limbs between the ankles and midthighs, and between the wrists and mid-upper arms. Pigmentation abnormalities and flexion contractures may also occur. NFD tends to affect the middle-aged population. Patients have a history of variable renal disease. Some patients had a previous non-transplant-related vascular surgery. Because of the systemic nature of the disease a new name for the syndrome (dialysis-associated systemic fibrosis) has also been recently suggested.

There are many types and causes of scleroderma-like disorders.

Deposition of agents different from mucin may also cause scleroderma-like skin changes. One of the typical examples is in patients with amyloidosis, where amyloid deposition causes scleroderma-like skin changes.

A blood eosinophilia can be observed in certain scleroderma-like disorders. Diffuse fasciitis with eosinophilia (eosinophilic fasciitis) is characterized by swelling and woody induration of skin of the extremities. Sclerodactyly and facial involvement are absent. Flexion contractures develop. Focal collections of eosinophils, and blood eosinophilia are typical signs.

Some metabolic diseases may also cause scleroderma-like skin changes. Skin thickness, digital sclerosis and limited joint mobility may be occasionally seen in children with insulin-dependent diabetes mellitus (IDDM). Adults with non-insulin-dependent diabetes mellitus may also show scleroderma-like skin thickness. Skin changes are usually seen in patients with long-standing, severe, complicated, maturity onset diabetes mellitus.

Porphyria cutanea tarda type II is characterized by skin symptoms on areas of the skin exposed to sunlight, especially on the face, ears and backs of the hands. Chronic ulcerating lesions are present developing from blisters. Hyperpigmentation and hypertrichosis also occur. Localized scleroderma-like changes or SSc-like form appear and show skin histology almost identical to idiopathic scleroderma.

Bone marrow transplantation is often necessary in severe malignant hematological diseases including leukemias. Chronic graft-versus-host disease (GVHD) is the major late complication of long time survivors of bone marrow transplantation, and occurs in 30-50% of these patients. Skin involvement may be generalized or restricted to selected areas. Sclerodermatous chronic GVHD usually develops progressively. In the localized form, the proximal limbs and the trunk are affected. Over a period of several months causing widespread cutaneous and subcutaneous fibrosis may develop with contractures. Skin ulcers may appear.

Patients with progeroid syndromes are characterized by early aging. One of the typical diseases is Werner's syndrome. Premature aging, early atherosclerosis, increased risk of cancer and diabetes and other endocrine diseases appear. Consanguinity is often present, a bird-like or a mask-like appearance and a characteristic body contour (short stature with a stocky trunk and very thin extremities are present). Gray hair, alopecia, cataracts, osteoporosis, and scleroderma-like skin changes (atrophic skin, skin sclerosis, skin ulcer, hyperkeratosis, hyper- or hypopigmentation, subcutaneous calcinosis, and telangiectasia) are present.

Causes include toxins and drugs.

Scleroderma-like syndromes provoked by chemical agents include eosinophilia-myalgia syndrome, toxic oil syndrome, and vinyl-chloride disease. Silica dust, epoxy resins, and solvents have been also described as potential provoking factors of systemic sclerosis (SSc) or scleroderma-like disorders.

Certain drugs including cytostatics such as docetaxel (taxotere), paclitaxel, gemcitabine, bleomycin, melphalan, and uracyl-tegafur may provoke scleroderma-like skin changes. These drugs are used for chemotherapy of malignant diseases. Appetite suppressants may also be scleroderma provoking agents. Certain local injections (corticosteroid, vitamin K, pentazocin) are also able to provoke scleroderma-like skin changes.

Physical injury including vibration stress is believed to provoke scleroderma. Four major complaints including Raynaud's phenomenon, numbness, coldness, and pain are usually present. Sclerodactyly may also be induced by vibration. Other physical effects, including limb immobilization, trauma, spinal cord injury, and radiation therapy may provoke systemic or localized scleroderma.

Table 1: Disorders with Scleroderma-like Skin Changes
Categories are not mutually exclusive.

❑**Amyloid Deposition**

❑**Chronic Graft-Versus-Host Disease (cGVHD)**

❑**Drug and Chemically-Induced**
- ❑ Appetite suppressants
- ❑ Cytostatic medications
- ❑ Eosinophilia-myalgia syndrome (EMS)
- ❑ Solvent-induced scleroderma
- ❑ Toxic oil syndrome (TOS)
- ❑ Vinyl chloride disease

❑**Endocrine Abnormalities**
- ❑ Diabetes
- ❑ Hypo/hyperthyroidism
- ❑ POEMS syndrome
- ❑ Progeroid syndromes

❑**Eosinophilia**
- ❑ Diffuse Fasciitis with eosinophilia (EF)
- ❑ Eosinophilia-myalgia syndrome (EMS)
- ❑ Scleromyxedema
- ❑ Toxic oil syndrome (TOS)

❑**Hereditary**

Early Aging:
- ❑ Progeroid syndromes (Werner's syndrome, etc.)

Skin Tightening or Atrophy:
- ❑ Atrophoderma of Pasini-Pierini
- ❑ Scleroatrophic and keratotic dermatosis of limbs (Huriez syndrome)
- ❑ Restrictive dermopathy

Skin Thickening:
- ❑ Melorheosthosis
- ❑ Phenylketonuria (PKU)
- ❑ Porphyria
- ❑ Stiff skin syndrome

❑**Metabolic/Biochemical Abnormalities**
- ❑ Carcinoid syndrome
- ❑ Diabetes Mellitus
- ❑ Hypothyroidism
- ❑ Nephrogenic fibrosing dermopathy
- ❑ Phenylketonuria (PKU)
- ❑ Porphyria

❏Monoclonal Gammopathy
- ❏ Myeloma with scleroderma-like skin changes
- ❏ POEMS syndrome
- ❏ Scleredema (occasionally)
- ❏ Scleromyxedema

❏Mucin Deposition
- ❏ Nephrogenic fibrosing dermopathy
- ❏ Scleredema
- ❏ Scleromyxedema
- ❏ Thyroid disorders

❏Physical Injury
- ❏ Radiation
- ❏ Trauma
- ❏ Vibration stress

◆ ❖ ◆

CHAPTER 2

Systemic Scleroderma
Caregiver Stories

To all who suffer from this,
my heart goes out to you.
You have strength bigger
than the world.
—Sunshine

Introduction to Caregiver Stories
by Carol Langenfeld, MSEd, PC, NCC

Carol Langenfeld is a professional counselor who has lived with scleroderma since 1977 and also has the experience of being a caregiver for her husband Doug during his long-time illness. They co-authored a book sharing the lessons they learned called Living Better: Every Patient's Guide to Living with Illness. Carol is a National Certified Counselor and a Licensed Professional Counselor in the State of Ohio.

"How do you do it?"

That question is frequently directed to patients and family caregivers. "We just had to find a new normal," replied a friend whose wife was in declining health from a long bout with lupus. This chapter gives us a glimpse of "new normal" for a variety of wonderful caregivers.

"New normal" looks different for every person who shares in another's illness as a caregiver. Caregivers wear many hats and demonstrate some key characteristics such as caring, advocacy, communication, perserverance, and self-awareness.

CARING. Caregivers show that they care in so many ways. Personalities are different. Each caregiver's relationship with the patient is unique. Some work outside their home, others are full-time caregivers. Some are healthy while many are dealing with their own health issues. Some caregivers are dealing with something totally new and unfamiliar while others have many years of experience. But whatever the circumstances, caregivers are caring people—caring the best they can under often difficult circumstances.

ADVOCACY. Every patient needs an advocate, one who stands up for their needs when they are not able or choose not to. Depending on the circumstances, a patient may be a very effective self-advocate. Other times, a patient needs a trusted caregiver to take on that role. An advocate learns what questions to ask and searches for medical answers. Sometimes, this may mean attending doctor appointments with patients, helping them with the job of paying medical bills, sorting out insurance claims, and helping deal with other business matters.

COMMUNICATION. Patients need someone who communicates with them. They need to be heard. Hearing and then communicating back what has been heard is not easy. To hear, stop talking out loud and stop the incessant brain dialogue humans carry on in their busy minds. To then communicate to the patient that they have been heard requires the caregiver to reflect back the patient's words so the patient knows they have been heard. If a patient asks for something that cannot be done, it is best to acknowledge this to keep their expectations in check.

PERSEVERANCE. This is perhaps the most difficult virtue of aiding someone with a long-term illness. Days and weeks of needs, aches, and pains become a year and then often many years. Patience, persistence, and positive personality are all important attributes to promote perseverance. But to persevere, one must also have the next characteristic as well.

SELF-AWARENESS. Caregivers often do many things that seem super-human to those looking in from the outside, but they are indeed human. Caregivers need to take care of themselves, too. Awareness of one's own need for assistance, connection, encouragement, time off, recreation, sleep, exercise, and nutrition is crucial. Support groups, both formal and informal, are essential for many caregivers. Airlines instruct passengers to put on their own oxygen mask first, before attempting to assist children with theirs. Caregivers must remember to do the same.

Readers will see many of the characteristics described above in the following stories by caregivers. Read their stories, share in their wisdom, and find encouragement in knowing that others have found the energy and resourcefulness to fulfill the challenging responsibilities of a caregiver.

Gerald Borntrager
Nevada, USA

"Gerry, something is not right. We need to go home."

It was Friday, January 2, 2004. It usually takes a lot to pull Sharon from her video poker games and live music at the Orleans Casino piano bar, but we left since she said she had to go home. The next day we were supposed to leave for San Diego so she could be with our daughter Amy and help her out in the final days of her pregnancy.

Sharon has always been one to get hit with colds and flu bugs worse then anyone in our family, but this time it seemed even more so. I asked some people at work if they could recommend a good doctor (we had tried others since we moved to Las Vegas and Sharon was not impressed by them) and Marsha in the accounting department recommended her doctor. I called him and was able to get an appointment for Sharon the next day. We figured we would just get some antibiotics and be done with it. Sharon was impressed, however, because he asked quite a few questions and wrote everything down. He gave us a prescription and ordered a chest X ray because of his concern with her shortness of breath. The diagnostics center was just down the street. We went there after leaving the doctor's office, stopped off to pick up the antibiotics, and went home so she could get back to bed. Early that same morning Amy gave birth to a healthy grandson, JD.

For years we knew something was wrong with Sharon. In my mind, it seemed to start back in the summer of 1988 while she was working and planting flowerbeds in Minnesota and suffered a heat stroke that landed her in the hospital. Shortly thereafter she had carpel tunnel surgery, and she developed Raynaud's in her hands.

She started seeing a rheumatologist. He mentioned connective tissue disease, but he did not put any particular name to it, or if he did, she did not write it down. She was taking medications for arthritis and for the blood circulation to her hands and feet. Then the heartburn started. While we lived in Minnesota, she had her esophagus scoped and stretched once, and told of the dangers of Barrett's esophagus. More drugs were prescribed for the acid reflux.

For years we had talked about moving south to get away from the cold. I was just getting sick of the winters, but for Sharon, we believed it was a matter of survival. Our youngest, Amy, graduated from high school in 2001, so the three of us made the move, leaving family and friends behind. It was about a year after we moved that Sharon started losing weight as she was once again having problems with swallowing and with irritable bowel syndrome. Another scope and stretch, and she was eating again. I guess Sharon and I both knew something was wrong. It seemed like every time we turned around something else was going wrong with her body. She often said she wished they could figure out what was wrong and give her the pill to fix it.

In late fall of last year, we went to the dentist because the nerves of some of Sharon's teeth started to become exposed. The dentist sent us to a periodontist, who in turn said before he could do anything, she would have to see a doctor about getting a physical. He was concerned for her dry mouth that had pretty much destroyed her taste buds and was causing the receding gum line. He thought it could be diabetes, but he admitted it was only a guess. So Sharon told her doctor, along with all her other ailments she had had over the years, and he took notes. The next day, he called Sharon and told her about his findings. Sharon was still pretty groggy when he called, but she was able to tell me that the doctor had found in his medical book something called CREST syndrome, and some other word that she did not write down. He said he had seen her chest X ray and had some concerns. He wanted blood tests, breathing tests, and an echocardiogram.

After dinner, I went to the computer and searched the Internet for CREST syndrome. I could not believe what I was reading. It was as if they were talking about Sharon on each web site. I asked Sharon, who was still feeling pretty sick and was in bed, if the doctor had mentioned systemic sclerosis. She said it didn't sound familiar, so I let her get back to sleep. Then I printed some of the web pages and left them on the table for her. The next day when I came home from work, Sharon was in tears. She said that the word her doctor used was scleroderma, which was also all over the papers I had printed the night before. She pointed out to me the parts on lung involvement, which indicated the latter stages of the disease. We had finally found the cause for all her ailments over all these years, only to find that there was no pill to make it better.

That Friday I took her in for the blood tests. Sharon said that she had never had so much blood taken for testing. The next week was the trip to the heart specialist. When he brought me in with Sharon to talk about the ultrasound pictures, at first he said everything looked fine, until we mentioned scleroderma. At that point he made sure to get an appointment set up for February 18. He talked about setting up a baseline for future visits.

We were supposed to go in for her lung capacity tests at the end of January, however Sharon had a flare so they put off the tests until February 19. But since we were there, I asked the main question, "Did the blood tests tell us anything? Is she officially diagnosed with scleroderma?" He showed us the blood report which stated "consistent with scleroderma." It was now official, although Sharon and I knew it already.

Yesterday was February 18th, Sharon's forty-fifth birthday, and the second visit to the heart specialist. After the tests, Sharon was told that the right side of her heart was enlarged, which is "consistent with someone with her condition."

Today we went in for her lung capacity test. Sharon said she should have practiced for it, that she could have done better. She just about passed out emptying her lungs into that machine, especially trying not to cough. Then came the medication, followed by another capacity check. The nurse made it sound like everything went well. But when Sharon's primary doctor came in to talk to us, we could tell right away he was uncomfortable. He told us that the tests indicated massive blockage, and even with the medication they applied, the results did not improve.

I got the impression he was ready for us to start pleading with him for some sort of relief for her, but both Sharon and I had been reading the literature, and knew what he was talking about.

This Saturday will be our first support group meeting. We are both wondering what to expect, but at least we will be able to talk to people who know what is going on with us. And next month we will be seeing a rheumatologist who is supposed to be able to handle scleroderma patients. So we will see if she has anything to help Sharon's constant coughing and the other pains associated with this disease. Of course, we pray she will make it to the appointment. This thing seems to be progressing rapidly.

Update – April 2004

Things have been pretty eventful since I last wrote. Within a week of Sharon's birthday, her breathing became very labored, and she ended up in the hospital for a week with pneumonia. Her heart specialist softly scolded her, saying that if she ends up with a fever and difficult breathing again, to get in right away. The way he put it, her lungs should be taking in four liters of air, but her disease has her limited to two liters, and she could take another half a liter off due to the pneumonia. Her newly assigned pulmonologist was also pushing for oxygen therapy after her stay, but she somehow managed to get out without it.

The next month included an angiogram, a sectional CT scan, a twenty-four-hour urine test, and numerous blood tests. She has about a half dozen different prescriptions that she is taking for circulation, high blood pressure, and indigestion, along with using nitroglycerin paste to help dilate the blood vessels in her hands.

Then came the first visit to the pulmonologist since she was in the hospital. Like everyone else, he asked her how long she had been smoking, which she answered with her usual, "Never have." He looked at the sectional CT scan and then checked her oxygen level with a finger monitor. He showed us on the X rays what pulmonary fibrosis looked like, and how far it had advanced. He started to talk about taking biopsies, but I think we talked him out of that idea. What was it going to tell us, that yes, she had fibrosis? He gave us the old "wait and see." But Sharon was not happy at all when he prescribed full time oxygen therapy, and scheduled it to be set up in our home that afternoon.

She has been on oxygen for about a month now, and she does admit it has helped her energy level. She has gotten over the stares of people who see her with the tank dolly. Just last week she was tested for using a pulse regulator, which allows her to use a smaller tank that she can carry. It is still a bother, but at least she does not have to use the tank dolly.

Sharon also has been having problems with swelling in her legs and feet. Her heart doctor prescribed a double dose of diuretics, along with potassium, and it seems to help, but she still has her bad days.

We have another support group meeting this weekend. We missed the one last month due to our moving Amy and JD into the house. Our son-in-law is in the Navy and will be deployed out to sea for six to eight months, and the timing worked well. It is nice having someone at home with Sharon, and, of course, Amy does want to be with her mom and JD (who is a real cutey).

Sharon still likes to hang out up at the Orleans, though we do not stay out as long as we used too. All of her friends have been very concerned and supportive, and if anyone asks, she tells them the oxygen is a temporary thing. But she does hide a lot of pain, which she tells me about but keeps from the outside world.

Update – September 2004

Since I last updated, things have not gotten any better.

In May, Sharon ended up in the hospital when her local lung doctor accidentally punctured her lung while trying to take a biopsy. When we went to see him in a follow-up visit, he came out and asked her if she was on oxygen at home, and he is the one who prescribed it! We have since changed our lung doctor.

We started going to see the specialists at UCLA. We saw Dr. Furst, one of the country's top scleroderma doctors, along with doctors in the pulmonology department. They ordered an echocardiogram with bubble study to be done of her heart, which we were able to have done here in Las Vegas. When we went in to have it done, Sharon ended up with a transient ischemic attack (TIA), which is a slight stroke, and ended up in the hospital overnight. A CAT scan showed that she had previously had a stroke, and the bubble study indicated a patent foramen ovale (PFO), which means there was a hole between the halves of her heart. Sharon's younger sister, Becky, had a TIA about two years ago, and ended up having a PFO closure device installed intravenously. This is also what the UCLA doctors suggested.

At the beginning of August, Sharon was in the hospital again with pneumonia. We had just seen her cardiologist earlier that day and she appeared fine. We told him about the flu shot she had just received, and he warned us that the shot would only protect her from certain strains, and that we still needed to be careful. That same evening, her temperature soared, and we drove her to the hospital. You should have seen the look on the doctor's face when he visited her in the hospital the next day! We all knew he did not have anything to do with her getting sick, but he felt awful for bringing up the possibility. He did point out how quickly things can change with her illness, and that we were right to get her to the hospital as soon as possible.

We also discussed the PFO closure with Dr. Leo, who immediately thought it was a bad idea. With her pulmonary hypertension, he told us that the PFO is something of a pressure relief valve, and that to close it in her could be devastating. We told him that before anything was done, they would need his approval, which they received after some phone calls and reassurances.

The day after Labor Day, we left for Los Angeles. The PFO closure was set for Thursday, but we had to have it done a day before so they could insert a catheter for medication to lower her pulmonary blood pressure. But because of her fibrosis, the pulmonary blood pressure remained high no matter what drugs they used. Her stay in the hospital changed from installing a PFO closure to examining her to see if she would qualify for a lung transplant. She had some morning fevers that alarmed the doctors, and she had another TIA, so she ended up staying two days longer than planned.

We are waiting for official notice from the UCLA transplant program, although from conversations we had with her doctors, we do not have our hopes up. Her stay in the hospital took its toll, leaving her drained.

She is slowly starting to get her energy back. We saw her rheumatologist the day after we returned. She reviewed Sharon's new drugs with her, and wrote a prescription for a wheelchair and a bathtub transfer bench.

When we were in the hospital waiting room with her second bout of pneumonia, Sharon laid the big one on me by saying, "If anything happens to me, do not let them bring me back." Talk about a hit in the stomach. But, with all that she has been going through and the pain that she is in, can I really blame her for the request?

I have one of two wishes, the first being that this terrible disease somehow reverses itself. The second would be that she suffers no pain, if my first wish is not granted.

◆ ❖ ◆

Karen Toneguzzi
Canada

Where do I start? Over the last year my mother has gone downhill rapidly from progressive systemic scleroderma. She has her throat stretched on a regular basis due to the tightening of the esophagus. She has been in and out of the hospital.

January 2003 started off terrible. Mom had been admitted to the hospital for a bowel obstruction, which was a common occurrence for her. She ended up staying for nineteen days. During this time, yet another specialist came to see her, suggesting she undergo a surgical procedure where a tube is inserted into the bowel to drain the obstruction. She was all set to do this when she developed a blood clot in her leg, from her thigh right down to her toes, so to this day she takes blood-thinning medication. Needless to say, her surgery was put on hold.

Her diarrhea is excessive, going twenty-five or more times in twenty-four hours. This was draining the life out of her, and her weight went down to eighty pounds, give or take a few. She could not walk down the hall to the bathroom anymore, so she needed to wear diapers.

Eventually her doctor said it was time to begin total parenteral nutrition (TPN), which is tubal feeding. We all knew she would end up needing TPN, but it was scary to hear this since all of us thought a feeding tube would mean it was the being the beginning of the end.

My mom has always been an active, vibrant woman, full of life, but this terrible debilitating disease sucked all that from her. But it did not take away her spirit. Her low blood pressure leaves her with very little or no strength. Her skin basically hangs on her bones. She is fragile to say the least.

The last straw came six weeks ago. We all gathered at my parents' house as she was going to be admitted the next morning for the insertion of the feeding tube. She could not even lift her head up from the couch to say hello to her four grandchildren. It turned out she had been bleeding internally, likely from the esophagus. The doctors figure that her esophagus had probably been scratched by violent vomiting that was caused by the bowel obstruction.

In the hospital, she had a blood transfusion, and she seemed to be getting better. On Good Friday, we almost lost her. Her body was drained of magnesium and calcium. They say she had fallen asleep, and likely she would have never woken up if my dad had not made the nurses call in a doctor. Thankfully, the doctor picked up on the problem through some blood tests and she pulled through.

Mom and dad were taken by air ambulance to Toronto General Hospital. She now has her TPN and she is home with us. It does not look scary, and it is not the beginning of the end; instead, it is a new beginning for her. She still faces the gastro-tube surgery, which perhaps will be done by the end of the summer. But we will take it one day at a time.

I remember my mom saying to me one night, "I am not going anywhere; I still have things to do." She was right. The team of doctors in Toronto have given us back our mother. She has gained an amazing twenty to twenty-five pounds, and still has a way to go, but at least she is here. Every day is a new day, a stronger day.

My mom is our hero. She is only fifty-nine years young. She has many more years ahead of her. And my dad is our hero for taking such good care of her. He is her main caregiver, her soul mate, her husband, and a wonderful father.

This disease is a terrible, devastating disease that has no boundaries. I love you, mom.

Khayriyyah Salaam
Alabama, USA

In August 2001, my daughter was living in Germany with her husband and two girls, who were four years old and seven months old. She began calling me with concerns of swollen hands that had a bluish hue. I am a registered nurse, so I immediately suspected Raynaud's syndrome and possibly lupus. I encouraged my daughter to go to a physician for a complete checkup.

After four months of military emergency room visits for joint pain, generalized weakness and malaise, we were exasperated and frustrated due to an inability to diagnose the problem.

In January 2002, my daughter was finally referred to a rheumatologist. The doctor took one look at my daughter and told her that she had scleroderma. The doctor immediately prescribed an ace inhibitor that helps to control blood pressure and subsequently protects the kidneys from the disease. The doctor in Germany also had my daughter shipped home because the severely cold winters in Germany are contraindicated for patients with scleroderma.

From that time until now, scleroderma has dictated our lives. The disease has attacked all the lobes of her right lung. All of her skin is affected, as are her joints. She is constantly in pain and has to take strong pain medication. She has contractures of both arms and legs. We are now trying to heal an ulcer on her coccyx. She has been hospitalized for pneumonia, acute renal failure, pancreatitis and upper bowel obstruction.

I praise God for his infinite mercy because she has recuperated from all of the conditions for which she was hospitalized. We take each day one day at a time with constant prayer and faith.

◆ ❖ ◆

Lancia
Italy

Some time ago a beloved friend of mine was diagnosed with scleroderma.

Everything started from the fact that she has a finger that was always cold and pale. She was taken to Modena and underwent an intervention. I do not remember the technical term, but it consists of unblocking the blood vessels. On this occasion she was diagnosed with scleroderma.

I wonder now if there is any relationship between the intervention she went through and the diagnosed disease?

Morgan Thomas
Ohio, USA

My mother has scleroderma. She was diagnosed last year. When she first noticed her symptoms, her lips were swelling and so were her eyes. Her friend told her she was around the age where she might have lupus, so she went to get tested for it.

Her doctor said that he thought she might have scleroderma. He then sent her to many doctors in different cities. Eventually she went to the Cleveland Clinic where she was diagnosed with scleroderma. She did not really know what it was, so the doctor kind of filled her in by telling her that it was a disease that turns you into stone. He told her a little more about it and then when she came home she told me.

I did not really know what it was and I got really scared. My mom told me that some people have died from the disease. I still get worried when I see her in the morning and she is all puffy. Her eyes are always swollen shut and her hands will not even close.

She went on disability and has a lot of trouble moving. She takes about twelve pills a day and I am concerned that it is too much medication.

I wish I could help her get rid of this disease, but all I can do is help her through it. I would like to hear from other people who are going through the same thing as my mother. I would also like to have answers to these questions:

1. Can you really die from this disease?
2. How many people have scleroderma?
3. Has anyone ever taken any medicine to help them through it and beat it?
4. Is there a possibility you can take too much medicine?

◆ ❖ ◆

Sunshine
Canada

It is heartbreaking to see the pain my mom suffers from this disease. I pray every day that a cure comes. I wish there was something I could give to her from my healthy body. If I could, I would do it in a heartbeat.

Her terrible scleroderma disease started with eating problems. It then proceeded into circulation problems, with cold hands and feet. Her hands would turn purple from being so cold.

Years later, she began suffering from painful ulcers on her hands, fingers, legs which would last for years. She was hospitalized. She was also in a wheelchair due to the excessive pain of the ulcers in her legs and feet. She had a homecare nurse for a few years. Now her ulcers are finally healing, but when one goes away, she gets another. Her pain is terrible.

She is such a trooper though. She pushes onward and acts as if she is in no pain at all. But her family knows better.

She is my hero. I wish for a cure every day. My biggest Christmas wish is not for presents, but for her to be all better.

To all who suffer from this, my heart goes out to you. You have strength bigger than the world.

Walter L. Ferguson
Virginia, USA

My name is Walter Ferguson. My son, Wally, was recently diagnosed as having scleroderma. I am sharing my story to help in any way I can toward finding a cure for this disease and better treatment of its adverse effects.

Wally is twenty-seven years of age. He is a CPA auditor for a major accounting firm. He got married this past June, and he and wife Megan, purchased a home a few months later. In November he received his diagnosis of scleroderma. He is the best son a father could ever hope to have.

His symptoms include his hands changing color in response to cold (Raynaud's), with ulcers beginning on the tips of his fingers. He has had Raynaud's for over a year. He is awaiting results of tests on effects of the disease on his kidneys and lungs. He is taking a circulation medication once a day and another medication to try to slow the buildup of collagen. He has been advised to wear gloves to keep his hands warm. His first visit was to a dermatologist, who sent him to a local rheumatologist for his current tests and treatment.

According to what I have read on the web, the cause of scleroderma is not known and at present, there are no drugs approved by the FDA or that have been adequately demonstrated by clinical study to modify the course of scleroderma.

Wally has always been strong and healthy. My wife and I need help in helping him cope with this terrible disease. We are reading a book written by Dr. Maureen Mayes, *The Scleroderma Book*, which is helpful.

We would appreciate any help and guidance offered to help in finding a cure and successful treatment, and in coping with this disease.

◆ ❖ ◆

Wes Coleman
West Virginia, USA

Just days ago, my sister Michelle was diagnosed with systemic sclerosis after being misdiagnosed for almost two years. She has all but one of the top ten symptoms. We will know in a few weeks if it has affected her organs or not.

Her symptoms started in her arms and hands, which led the first doctor to diagnose carpal tunnel, considering only the fact that she types a lot at work. It then left her hands and arms for awhile, and started to affect her hips and legs. But, the doctor still proclaimed that it was carpal tunnel.

Shortly after that, she had trouble grasping the simplest of objects, and tying her shoelaces. She then decided to seek out a more intelligent doctor. This new doctor seemed to think that she may have lupus, which is a common misdiagnosis for scleroderma. Thankfully, this caused her to get on the right track with treatments.

I had never even heard of scleroderma until a few days ago when my sister called me and broke the horrible news to me. I did not quite understand that this was serious until I found it on the Internet. Then I broke down and cried like a three-year-old.

She is only twenty-eight years young and I am only thirty. I have epilepsy, and now she has this. How much more can two 'kids' take? She has only been married for a few years and has a young son to take care of. I feel guilty because I live over one hundred miles away and cannot be there for her every day.

In the stories that I have read, it sounds like it takes years to develop all of the symptoms. Michelle has developed almost all of them in less than eighteen months.

I am not trying to dump on anyone; I just need to vent and maybe let some other sibling know that they are not alone when dealing with this terrible disease when it has struck someone that you love.

Every day I wish that I could take her pain away and make it my own. I do not understand how something so awful could happen to someone so special who is just learning what life and love are all about!

Update – April 2004

When I left my story back in January, I was still ignorant about this horrible disease. I have since learned a great deal about scleroderma. I am not saying that I am coping any easier; I just understand more of what is going on with my sister.

Last month, her doctor finally sent her to Pittsburgh, Pennsylvania, where she met with one of the best doctors in the world for this illness. I am sorry that I cannot remember his name, but if anyone would like, I can ask my sister and would be more than happy to send it to them.

Michelle told me that he treated her like a human being who was trying to live life and not one who was making up symptoms to get attention. She sat in his office for several hours, not waiting on him, but actually talking to him! He explained to her exactly what she had, her options, and her chances.

Unfortunately, her options and chances are slim. He told her to not even think about having another child for three to five years, because in this time period her condition would most likely worsen. But, in the event that she does beat this, she would probably be in the clear after about five years; however, he was completely honest with her and told her that he did not foresee her improving anytime soon. He did tell her though, that she was in the best hands and that he would be there with her to help her in her fight!

My sister still has her good and bad days, mostly bad. She is still holding her job at the bank, still being the best mom to her son, and trying to be the wife her husband needs her to be. But, she has finally agreed to have someone come in and clean her house once a week. It is not much, but at least it is something!

So far, the disease has not spread to her organs but she and I both know that it is probably just a matter of time. We do not speak of the disease much anymore, probably because we know what the other is thinking, and we try not to dwell on the bad, we just concentrate on being there for each other and enjoying our time together, whether it is for three years or three hundred!

In today's world we often do not tell the ones we love, or even show them for that matter, just exactly how we feel, whether it is out of shame, fear of rejection, or whatever. I am not ashamed of the feelings that I have for my sister. She has been my rock through out the years and now it is my turn to finally repay her by being her rock!

I believe it is important to tell our family, friends, children, on a daily basis, that we love them, whether or not they are healthy. I thought my dad was in great health, and he passed away not knowing that I truly loved him. I will never get the chance to tell him how I felt.

Now, whenever I depart from a loved one, or say good-bye on the telephone, instead of saying, "I love you, good-bye!" I say, "Good-bye, I love you!" That way, if something terrible ever happens, our last word will not be, "Good-bye."

Since I posted my story back in January, I have heard from many people expressing their sorrow, asking questions, and lending their support. I want to thank each and every one for being here and sharing. I greatly appreciate it!

CHAPTER 3

Systemic Scleroderma Patient Stories

Do not give up! Fight the battle!
We may not win but we will not be
brought down that easily!"

—Naomi

Introduction: The Call of Challenge
When an Autoimmune Disease Presents Itself
by Judith R. Thompson Devlin

When an autoimmune disease presents itself, our first challenge is to get up every morning. Once we manage to do that regularly we are more able to meet the other, seemingly endless challenges of having a chronic illness.

Many of our lives were sideswiped by a diagnosis of an incurable disease in the prime of our lives. Many of us were given a 'deadline' of a few more years. Many of us have lived well past that initial time frame.

I remember being devastated when my doctor told me I may have five to seven more years after being diagnosed with CREST scleroderma in 1991. I calculated the months, documented the D-Day in my journal, and spent those years waiting to die and preparing myself and my daughter with hospice volunteer training. I got closer to my family and made amends with them. I became more peaceful and found joy and education in reading, including many books on the topic of dying. I was ready.

Then the morning after D-Day presented itself, I was still alive. Phew. But what should I do now? I had not thought much about a future beyond seven years, which was 1998.

For a few weeks I pondered my scleroderma, my living circumstances, and my life in general. I thought about all the things I had not done and still wanted to do.

There really was not much left to do, except for taking a hot air balloon ride (which my daughter gave me on my fiftieth birthday); having a successful relationship with a man (I got married in 2003 and am working on that, which is proving to be much tougher than living with scleroderma); owning my own home (which came with my marriage); kayaking (I love it! It is a great range-of-motion exercise, exhilarating, and I have had one white rapid close call); snowshoeing and golf (which also came with my marriage).

I wanted to keep writing and producing books (this is my sixth book), and I hoped to become a grandmother (I have a new grandson!). I even have a new cat, since my two other cats that were with me for eighteen years through what I thought were my last years, have both passed on.

I am really living again, not just existing as a disabled, chronically ill middle-aged woman. I have lost most of my hearing, which in many ways makes my life very peaceful. I have lost normal bowel control. This week I will lose all my teeth and get dentures. I have trouble walking since my feet have lost their natural padding. Occasionally I still want to stay in bed, but because of stiffness, aches and pain, that option is more painful than getting up for each new day. I have learned to ignore the chronic fatigue. I make it a point to watch the sunrise almost every morning from my deck in my hot tub, which helps with the stiffness and gives me the glorious joy of having a new day.

I have learned to meet my challenges head on. I am happy to still be alive. It has not been a piece of cake, but my scleroderma, though often difficult, has given me better coping skills to deal with life. Before I had scleroderma, I often ran away when life presented insurmountable problems. Now I stay, accepting and meeting my life challenges with zest and zeal! I now have character, dignity, a legacy and a real life.

Scleroderma has taught me how to live. When we listen to its lessons, we have a better life. Everything happens for a reason. By meeting our challenges with grace, humor, and an open heart and mind, nothing is impossible!

Brian D. Jessop
Utah, USA

Someone asked me for help on how to fight this scleroderma, and I said yes.

I am a Vietnam veteran who served from 1968 to 1970. I was there during the Agent Orange time on the Saigon River and the Macon Delta Rivers.

I am writing this because someone from Iran asked for help in finding someone who knows how to treat scleroderma. I know two people. One doctor is the head of the Dermatology Department at the University of Utah and the other doctor is at the Veterans Administration Hospital in Salt Lake City, Utah.

My doctor at the University of Utah finally diagnosed me after years of tests. I was sick of all the tests; I felt like I was a human test tube.

We tried radiation, and that worked for a short time. I was able to do things that I had not been able to do for over fifteen years, but it messed me up some. Now my mouth is very dry and I have to drink a lot of water. I was in so much pain that it was very hard for me to walk by the afternoon, so my doctor helped me obtain a scooter to ride when my feet would not work.

I went to many clinics around Utah. Over the years I spent over ten thousand dollars just trying to find out how to help myself. Then I found another doctor who is a total wellness chiropractic physician. He has helped me a lot. Before I met him I would get up every day and ask God to come and get me. Now after much physical therapy I feel much better, so I no longer ask God to come and get me. Instead I ask Him to help me each and every day. I am not out of the woods yet, but I am in better shape.

I get three massages a week. Two of them are a good workout and make me feel great, but the one in the middle of the week is a deep tissue massage and it is painful. I swim one to three times a week. I also do Qigong and yoga once a week. This is what I have found it takes for me to keep ahead of scleroderma.

A lot has happened to me and my health and it will be an uphill fight. But I am not willing to give this life up, so I will press on.

This year the Veteran's Administration in Salt Lake City started a new program. It is an optional eight week class called "Choosing to Heal" that has an integrative approach. It works with the Qigong class. It seems that when I take this class I have to watch my insulin closer because most of the time I need less insulin on those nights.

Some of the men I have talked to said this class did not do anything for them, but I am sick of being sick and I have to look for help all over the place. I am not ready to give up yet so I will do whatever it takes to make me feel better. Feeling better is good. I have been fighting scleroderma for fifteen years now and if I can answer any of your questions, I will do what I can.

The doctors behind this program have done a lot to help me move about. It has taken a lot of people to make it so I can walk and move again. I am still in pain, but if I take my medications, my feet, arms and the rest of my body say, "Go out and do your best."

Christy
Ohio, USA

On my fortieth birthday, I made the decision to pursue a business degree while working full time. I was feeling somewhat run down at the time and decided it was time to have a checkup. I went to my family physician who recommended I have my blood chemistry tested.

When I called their office for the results, the woman on the other end said I tested positive for lupus. This test result was devastating news until my family physician returned from vacation, called me and explained the test was not indicative of a positive lupus test, but rather high antinuclear antibody (ANA) levels, and recommended I see a specialist. I was diagnosed with systemic scleroderma. The symptoms I was experiencing pointed directly to CREST.

I began a regular schedule of routine visits twice a year. There was never enough time between visits or freedom from pain to let me forget the shadow that had cast itself upon me. I have tried to do everything humanly possible to outrun the shadow.

I just experienced my forty-eighth birthday. I will never forget the look on my daughter's, husband's and parents' faces when I graduated from school. Fortunately, I have been able to continue working. I firmly believe that if I slow down, I will lose momentum. However, I am more selective on what I consider quality time. Now, I have resigned myself to the fact that it is okay to sit outside in my herb garden or pet my dogs, and just let the housework go. Housework will always be there tomorrow. Special moments that give us true pleasures are sometimes too few and far between.

Most importantly, during these past eight years, I have turned to my faith. I have learned from personal experience that sometimes not even our closest friends want to hear about medical changes taking place within us. It is not because they do not care, but rather their fear of the shadow. My faith has taught me not to judge, but accept their friendship and make the most of each moment.

◆❖◆

Donna D. Munoz
California, USA

I am a fifty-nine-year-old female and I was diagnosed with systemic scleroderma three months ago.

At this time the problems are mostly skin-related, with hardening and lesions. I am tired a lot and am in pain under my arms. The back of my knees are so hard that I have difficulty bending. I am frequently chilled.

I am just beginning to have difficulty swallowing and have pain in my kidney area.

My legs do not straighten out in bed at night due to swelling in the groin area and tightening of the skin. I seem puffy. I do not have the typical involvement in my hands and it took months and many tests to diagnose my case.

No one shares a timeline with me or will tell me what to expect next. I am trying to just enjoy each new day and attack each new symptom as it comes about.

Kathy
Florida, USA

In 1994 I was hospitalized with my blood pressure going through the roof; my systolic pressure was over three hundred!

I was in intensive care for two weeks and the doctors were unable to tell me why my blood pressure had soared so high. They felt at one time there was a blockage going into my kidneys. They did a catheterization and found nothing.

After three weeks of being in the hospital, I was released with no diagnosis. I felt so weak, just walking from my kitchen to the living room exhausted me. I was sent to a nephrologist (a kidney doctor) and he diagnosed me with hypothyroidism. Nothing new was discussed.

In 1996 I got this hard piece of skin on the pointer finger of my right hand. This was very small, but painful. It really bothered me while bowling. I was given a name and telephone number for a local dermatologist and I went to see him.

He gave me this bandage-thing and told me to put it on during the day and take it off at night. When I took it off, it took a wad of skin from my finger. Within two weeks the end of my finger was so sore that when I bumped it, it took my breath away.

At my second appointment with the dermatologist, he was quite worried. He explained to me this looked like a finger ulcer due to scleroderma. I had never heard of this before. He sent to a pain management doctor. The next thing I knew, he was doing nerve blocks on me three times a week. This made life almost impossible, since I could not work and my mother had to take me in for the treatments. After a month of these blocks, only one or two treatments actually worked, and I had had enough. I demanded to have the finger taken off, and I found a surgeon who did remove the tip of my finger.

The doctor who had been doing the nerve blocks had told me I had scleroderma, but never mentioned that I needed to see a rheumatologist. He never told me to keep my hands warm to ease the pain. He told me nothing except just come back for more nerve blocks and take heavy pain medications, antidepressants, and pills to help me get up and go. I was very very lucky to not become addicted to any of these drugs.

I then found some information on the Internet about scleroderma. Several sites said most people die within ten years of being diagnosed, the pain was unmanageable, and it would be a painful death. I was thirty-seven at the time and I thought my life was over.

I made an appointment with a rheumatologist and he was nice enough to straighten it all out for me. I am now forty-three. I still get painful finger ulcers, and I just recently had a heart attack. No one can tell me if the heart attack had anything to do with the scleroderma.

There could have been more details to my story, but it hurts my fingers to type. I hope this story helps someone, now or in the future.

Naomi
New Jersey, USA

Hi, my name is Naomi. In 1985 I became pregnant with my fourth child. After carrying the baby for five months, I suddenly began to bleed. I immediately called my doctor and was told to go into the office. After several tests they told me my baby was fine. A week later my baby was dead. Later I found out that my baby had never developed in my body; I was five months pregnant but the baby was the size of a one-month pregnancy and therefore could not survive. Thus began my problems.

Several months later I began to experience cold hands and feet with blue hands and sores on my fingers. I believe this was the beginning of my illness, although I was not diagnosed with scleroderma until 1991! To top it off I had the worst kind, systemic sclerosis. The specialist that saw me was very good and did not beat around the bush. I will never forget her words to me. She looked me in the eyes and said to me and my husband that scleroderma was a disease which had no cure and no medications, other than experimental ones.

I asked her the prognosis and she said, "Two years." I looked at her in utter disbelief! My life flashed in front of me. Here I was in my early thirties with three little children at home and this doctor is telling me that within two years I could be dead. I looked at her and I remember telling her that there was no way I was going to die! I had children to raise.

Well, guess what? That was thirteen years ago! Not only did I raise my children but on October 4th and then again on November 1st of this year, I married off my two boys.

I made it through their graduations and also through their weddings. They were so grateful to be able to dance the 'son and mother dance' at their wedding that they (and me along with the guests) cried through the whole song. And I have no plans of going anywhere. I will fight this battle until my body cannot take it any more. My doctor is astonished by my attitude, considering I have Raynaud's, my fingers are curling up, I have lost my nails, and I have pulmonary fibrosis, acid reflux, aspergillosis and an irregular heart. I am on oxygen all the time, and can only walk a short distance. Because my left lung collapsed due to so much scar tissue, I have partially lost my voice.

But I have faith, which gives me the strength to continue on. I look forward to hopefully having grandchildren some day so I plan to be around for a while longer.

It is true that I have more bad days then good ones but I am thankful every day I am alive. I have also inspired others who suffer from other kinds of illnesses. I encourage them to fight and not to give up. And I encourage all readers to do the same.

Do not give up! Fight the battle! We may not win but we will not be brought down that easily!

Denise
New Jersey, USA

My name is Denise and I am forty-three years old. I was first diagnosed with diffuse scleroderma in February 2002, but my symptoms began subtly in the summer of 2000.

It started off with swollen hands and feet. My rings no longer fit and some of my shoes were tight. At first I wrote it off to water retention from premenstrual syndrome (PMS). Then in early fall I had bad carpal tunnel syndrome and ended up having surgery in December. The hand surgeon suggested I see a few specialists since swollen fingers are not a symptom of carpal tunnel. Also, certain autoimmune diseases can cause carpal tunnel syndrome.

That winter I developed Raynaud's in my hands and feet and went to see a rheumatologist. I saw her a few times and she kept saying that it was only Raynaud's and that ten percent of the population have it. But I was not convinced, since the skin on my fingers appeared different to me, and my fingers were still swollen. I sought a second opinion, and it did not take the doctor long to suspect scleroderma. This doctor referred me to a rheumatologist who specialized in scleroderma.

I was lucky to get in to see him after a three month wait. After this rheumatologist thoroughly examined me, he put it all together and diagnosed me with diffuse systemic sclerosis.

It took almost two years to come to this diagnosis, and it probably would have taken longer if I had not educated myself about the disease and suspected something more than Raynaud's early on. If you feel there is something wrong and you know you are not a hypochondriac, then please take the initiative and do not give up until you are satisfied and have an answer.

This takes me to where I am today, and I am doing rather well so far. I still see my doctor every few months, and my lungs get checked also. I was on a short course of medication last year, and it seems to have stopped or at least slowed the progression of the disease. My doctor is confident that it is no longer life-threatening, and I have faith in him since I feel he is one of the best. So I will try to believe that.

As of now, my Raynaud's seems to be worsening, so I do what I can to prevent getting an attack, such as carrying hand warmers in my coat pockets or pocketbook. I do this even in the warm weather due to air-conditioning. Raynaud's is a pain in itself; but oh, how I wish that my first rheumatologist had been right when she said that it was only Raynaud's!

I have the aches, pain, fatigue, depression, finger ulcers, swelling, and digestive problems that go along with the disease. Some days are worse than others. I try to take care of myself by exercising within my ability, which is one of the reasons I feel I am doing better than I would be otherwise. That is very important. I take vitamins, but I always have. I rest when needed and try not to overdo it. I listen to my body.

I do not work anymore because the unpredictability of this disease makes it very hard for me to hold a job. Not working also better enables me to take care of myself. I do not think I would be doing so well if I had the stress of holding a job and keeping a home and family. Truthfully, I wish I could work; but realistically I do not feel I can. I try to keep myself busy in between caring for myself and for my family.

I am learning all I can about this disease. Thank goodness for the Internet! I am trying to keep contact with various support groups online, as well as with meetings when I can. Unfortunately, there are not any support groups in my area, but we are working on it. I feel it is important to know that there are many others like us and many much worse, who suffer with this relatively rare disease.

I do not know what the future holds, so I am just living my life the best that I can.

Jewell
Canada

When I think back, I had been getting sick for a long time. I just did not know it. I put the fatigue, headaches, joint pain and body pain down to working too much.

For years I would be sick off and on but prided myself on not missing a day of work. However, I started doing a fair bit of contract work, which meant I would be working for anywhere from a day to eleven or more months. Increasingly, at the end of the contracts, I would just crash. Looking back, those were the taps on the shoulder I should have been paying attention to. Instead I just kept on going, sometimes work-sharing or working shorter contracts. The reality was, I loved my work and I think that helped me to stay in denial.

I then took a position where I would no longer be doing ongoing contract work all the time and I was in the midst of forming a consulting company with some friends before I got sick. This would mean taking contracts while still working a full-time job. We had just gotten our first big contract when I got sick. I cannot tell you how disappointed I was over this. I knew I was getting older and it was time to stay in one place and settle down some. However, I still wanted variety in what I did, and that is what I hoped having a consulting company would serve. Also, I would still have a position with regular hours as well as holidays and benefits.

Where I had prided myself on never missing a day of work from sickness, I now caught everything that was going around and for the first time ever I was not only missing days, I was missing many days, sometimes using up a lot of sick days. This was just not like me. I often felt awful but did not want to tell anyone as somehow I felt it made my life more vulnerable. I did not want someone telling me that it was time to find a new line of work.

One day in April 1996, I woke up and literally could not move. I phoned into the office and told them that and then said I would be there by the afternoon. I remember thinking about how much work I needed to get done. By the time the afternoon rolled around, I knew I would not be able to work and phoned into work again. To make a long story short, I did this for three days in a row before I knew I was not getting up at all for awhile.

I saw a dermatologist and a rheumatologist. I was diagnosed with chronic fatigue syndrome (CFS), fibromyalgia, and Raynaud's. At the time, I could not understand why I was not being diagnosed with lupus, as my symptoms were so like those I had heard of with lupus sufferers and I had positive antinuclear antibodies (ANA). I still believe I have a lupus overlap, but no one has agreed with that yet. Both of my doctors were very good, but one retired after I had been seeing him for some time and the other became ill with cancer. Unfortunately, it was time to look for another specialist.

In the meantime, I had been doing some research on the Internet and came across information on silicone breast implants and the illnesses attached to them. I had my implants shortly after nursing my last child, about twenty years prior. I became very interested in 1992 when the United States Food and Drug Administration banned breast implants, which had never actually been approved. The plastic surgeon told me that they would last forever and that I could even nurse a baby if I chose to. I was wondering then if I should get mine taken out, but when subsequent stories by the manufacturers came out denying the evidence, and women came out in groups using my buzz word, "choice," I thought that maybe I had been overreacting as well. I certainly did not want to lose my breasts, so I comfortably drifted into denial.

Then, I came across one web site that mentioned the symptoms most of the affected women were having. After seeing the symptoms all listed at one time like that and being only too acquainted with my own symptoms, my jaw dropped and I found myself sobbing for the first time since I had become ill. I had far more symptoms than what I saw on that page, and all but three of the symptoms listed.

I went to see another specialist who was experienced with breast implants. In addition to what I had already been diagnosed with, he diagnosed me with a particular kind of arthritis called arthropathy. I had it pretty much throughout my whole body, including my backbone and my breastbone. He also diagnosed me with Sjögren's syndrome, irritable bowel syndrome (IBS) and gastro-esophageal reflux disease. I had a bone density exam that showed I also have osteoporosis as a result of having had a complete hysterectomy in my early thirties. My symptoms never went away though, and now I see the hysterectomy as being completely unnecessary.

Before this, a doctor who I saw for a short time diagnosed me with emphysema. I did not believe it. In fact, at the time, I thought he was just trying to get me to quit smoking. I was a fool. Since then I have been diagnosed with chronic obstructive pulmonary disease (COPD). I smoked for thirty-six years and quit about two and a half years ago.

Around the time I had my breast implants removed, the skin on my hands, arms, shoulders, chest, face, back, legs, hips, buttocks, sides, ribs and stomach became, itchy, inflamed, bloody in places from scratching, and hard. By that time, I had been so downtrodden by illness, questions and problems with an insurance company, and just everything, that I did not even want to go to the doctor. My neighbor, who is an intensive care unit nurse, told me it was important to get it checked out.

I was sent to a dermatologist respected by my primary doctor, who has been wonderful throughout this process, and I cannot imagine going through all this without him. He took a look at my laboratory tests and history and just kept on asking question after question, not allowing me to swerve off even a little bit. At the end of his examination he told me that I have progressive systemic sclerosis of the diffuse variety. He said it was very serious, and that if I developed any other symptoms, I should jump up and down and scream until I got attention if I was not being taken seriously. He also said he was going to phone my primary doctor right then (whom I was on my way to see) and tell him how important this was, and recommended that I be referred to a highly regarded rheumatologist/internist.

I went to see him and he agreed with the diagnosis of the dermatologist, and also said the echocardiogram indicated that there is slight thickening on the pericardial sac of my heart and possible pericardial effusion. From there, he referred me back to the rheumatologist I had been seeing prior to him.

When I had the breast implants removed, sure enough, they were both ruptured. Calcinosis was found in the breast tissue, something that people with scleroderma know a lot about.

I have had esophageal and angina attacks that have landed me in the hospital. I am starting to get to know the difference between the two. I get these attacks at rest, so MIBI scans will not detect what is happening, as they rely on activity and stress on the heart. Both kinds of attacks respond to nitroglycerin. If I wear a nitroglycerin patch to bed at night, I get fewer attacks. This is the patch I am supposed to be wearing during the daytime, but the way I see it, I am more protected with my blood pressure medication then, and this method has significantly cut down the number of attacks for me. I also use nitroglycerin during the day if I feel something coming on. If I am woken up by one of the attacks, it is usually well along, much more painful, and much more scary.

Not that long ago I was put on a course of cyclophosphamide. My blood was being closely monitored during this time. I got a call from my rheumatologist at one point saying that he was concerned about my white blood cell count and suggested that I go off the cyclophosphamide for three days, and then start again at a lower dosage. That went on until the next blood tests came back, and my doctor phoned me again and wanted me to get in to see him as soon as possible. The problem was that I was too sick to go! In fact, I am often too sick to go to the doctor. That is why I build up my energy, so that I can make my doctors appointments! During that time my doctor was scared that my kidneys were going to fail.

It was ISN's Sherrill Knaggs who helped me throughout this period of time. I would have been so scared without her. We emailed each other back and forth as I went through my blood tests. Because Sherrill's kidneys had failed, she knew how to handle me. I say as often as I can, "Thank you, Sherrill." She held my hand throughout the whole, awful and scary ordeal. The ISN's Message Board has helped me immensely; the people are kind and knowledgeable. I keep on learning and feel as though I am even more up-to-date on the latest research than most doctors.

I find that the worst part about this disease is the unpredictability of the symptoms from day to day. The times in between are also hard, when you are nearing a new diagnostic part of the disease and the uncertainty of tests that may or may not detect something specific to scleroderma. For example, sometimes things do not show up on tests, yet you know something is wrong. Many doctors know very little about scleroderma, so we as patients have to really keep on top of what is happening regarding this disease through research and other people. That is why this forum of scleroderma patients from all over the world is so important! We keep ourselves well informed and well supported to boot! There is no cure yet, but by working together we can make it happen, if not for ourselves, for the younger people.

I think this forum is very important in advocating for and by helping each other. We learn enough to advocate on behalf of ourselves during these very uncertain times, although learning when and how to treat the disease is still somewhat of a mystery.

I wish I had known about the ISN web site at www.sclero.org long ago, because there is a lot of ambiguity in diagnosing autoimmune and/or connective tissue diseases. We know we belong here when what is happening to others is similar to our own story.

This site is a fine example of how technology should be working, with people all over the world helping other people with the same challenges. For those who are too ill to even make it on a continual basis to support groups, which are rare for such a rare disease, this is a wonderful alternative. Thank you, ISN!

From my research, I believe that my scleroderma was caused by silicone implants. I think that in the future, this idea will be as accepted as cigarettes causing cancer and asbestos causing asbestosis/cancer. The same public relations campaigns have been run with all of theses agents. There may be genetic predispositions, but how can we possibly be immune to all that poison?

I am glad to be part of this scleroderma community, because it has helped me so much! I am just not glad about the way I got here. I pray that silicone breast implants will not be allowed back on the market. If they are, I pray for the lives of the women they will impact.

❖❖❖

Judy Tarro
California, USA

The best we can figure, I was diagnosed with diffuse scleroderma in 1956. We did the usual "scleroderma shuffle" going from doctor to doctor trying to find out what was wrong with me. Eventually, my own doctor suspected scleroderma and recommended that I go to the medical center at the University of California Los Angeles (UCLA). It was there that the diagnosis of my illness was made.

Since then, Raynaud's, Sjögren's, pulmonary fibrosis, pulmonary hypertension, and thyroid problems have been added to the mix.

It is almost to the point that I am fearful of getting up in the morning, afraid that parts will start falling off. Yikes! Well, not really. I have known no other way of life, so I do not think living with scleroderma is all that unusual. I quite honestly do not know what normal is.

My lung involvement progressed to the point where I now need supplemental oxygen. Everywhere I go I have to tote around my "friend." It is not pleasant, but it is a necessity that I have gotten used to.

My parents treated me no differently than my sister. We did most things together, as much as I could, anyway. My parents were told I would not live beyond my teens. Hah! A lot they knew! Well, actually, they did not. There was not a whole lot of research being done then, so I suppose no one quite knew what to do with me.

There was no treatment back then, so I never really took anything for it except once, but I do not know what it was. My doctor sent for something that was in a clinical trial somewhere "back East." It was a powder that was mixed with glucose water and I was given intravenous treatments of this daily for three weeks. We did this twice, a few years apart. There is no way to tell if it did anything or not as scleroderma will go into remission on its own. But, as I went through my teens, the disease did back off somewhat.

From the beginning I was unable to do much physically. My joints tightened up and it was difficult for me to even get up from the floor. This sure took care of any aspirations I had of mountain climbing, if I had ever wanted to do such a thing. Besides, the cold on the mountains triggers Raynaud's attacks. Yuck. I never could play any sports, but that was okay with me. After graduation, I got a job and worked for many years.

Meanwhile the disease progressed. Eventually it got to be much more than I could handle, and I went on disability. That was fourteen years ago. I have been very busy, but, I do things in my own time, resting when I need it.

Right now I am working on a dollhouse. I never had one when I was a child. So I decided it was about time! I built one from a kit and built the furniture to go inside. Some of the furniture was from kits, but some was from my own design. I am also now working with polymer clay, making things for the dollhouse, gifts, whatever pops into my head.

I have my own personal web site, and with two other women I created SD World. It is a web site, email list and support group for folks with scleroderma or other autoimmune diseases. I am webmaster, so I am often busy upgrading and maintaining it. It allows me to put my feet up in the afternoons for awhile, too. Now there is a pleasant thought; I think I shall go do that right now!

Karen Russell
Michigan, USA

Hi, my name is Karen, also known as Pooh Bear, and I have diffuse scleroderma, fibromyalgia and Raynaud's. A number of years ago I began having some weird feelings on my left side. My face and arm would sort of feel like it was sleeping. My doctor ordered a CAT scan of the brain thinking it was a possible stroke, because I also have high blood pressure. The scan was normal and the doctor thought I may have had a transient ischemic attack (TIA) or mini stroke.

As time went on this feeling would come on more often. Then I started having trouble walking. I was sent to University of Michigan Medical Center where I was told I had arthritis in my back and a pinched nerve in my shoulder. This was in January of 2003. I had surgery on my shoulder and the tingling feeling seem to disappear for awhile.

But then other symptoms began. My fingers would get ice cold and turn pure white, almost transparent. My muscles seemed to ache all over. I felt like I had been hit by a truck. I would have good days and bad. I went to see a rheumatologist and she diagnosed me with fibromyalgia and Raynaud's. She said there was nothing that could be done for the fibromyalgia except to stay active and exercise to keep from becoming stiff.

Things sort of stayed the same for a few months. Then in October, my skin became real tight. I felt as though I was sunburned from head to toe. It hurt to be touched anywhere. If I stretched out my arm it felt as though my skin was going to rip.

I went back to my rheumatologist, and she diagnosed me with diffuse scleroderma. My daughter was with me at that visit. I was so glad she was there, because I sort of went into shock when the doctor said she was going to start me on chemotherapy treatments. When she explained what the disease could do and that there was no cure, I broke down. I thought I had been given a life sentence with no parole. She explained to me that the disease was a progressive one and that different people had different experiences.

I got myself together, and with my daughter, got on the Internet. The research enlightened me about the disease and its outlook for life expectancy. I made up my mind that I was going to beat this monster, no matter what. I know the road ahead is probably going to be tough, but so am I.

I had no bad side effects from the chemotherapy, other than being tired all the time. I was taking the treatments orally, every day. I never lost my hair or got sick.

In February, I went in for my monthly checkup and blood work. The doctor called me the next day and said my liver count was up. I was to take only one pill a day of the chemotherapy instead of two, and avoid alcohol and over-the-counter pain medications. I was to do this for two weeks and then have the blood work done again.

I did all this, but the next count was even higher. I was taken off the chemotherapy entirely for two more weeks and had blood work drawn again. The results were better. I am off the chemotherapy two more weeks and then I will have my blood drawn again on April 30th. We will see what happens. The doctor says I may have to have the chemotherapy given intravenously rather than orally. I guess too much chemotherapy is just as bad as none at all.

My fingers are starting to curl inward, so the doctor had splints made for both hands that I wear to bed at night to try to straighten them and keep them from getting worse.

My fingertips are very sensitive. I have not had any ulcers yet, thank goodness. I wear gloves whenever I do dishes, reach into the freezer, go outside, or do anything that could harm them. My Raynaud's is really bad.

My legs are getting weaker and quite painful. Like before, I have good days and bad. But even on the bad days I have my family. I have three fantastic children, ages sixteen, twenty-two, and twenty-four, and the best husband a woman could ask for. He is the greatest. So through it all, with God on my side and a terrific family, I am going to be just fine. God bless everyone who has to deal with this monster. My thoughts and prayers are with you. Together we will get it through it.

◆ ❖ ◆

Kim Curry
Pennsylvania, USA

I am a forty-two-year-old wife, mother of two sons (Dana, age twenty-five and Craig, age fourteen) and a granddaughter (Malea, who is eight months old). I work full-time, attend college parttime, and also work as the secretary of my church.

I was diagnosed in February 2002 with diffuse scleroderma. I also suffer from Raynaud's, Sjögren's Syndrome, a hiatal hernia, and polymyositis. I recently had pancreatitis and had to have my gall bladder removed after a severe attack.

My father, who died two weeks before my seventh birthday, had sickle cell anemia and I was born with sickle cell trait.

In October of 2000 my mother contracted a very bad case of pneumonia. She was hospitalized for three weeks and had another two to three months of recuperation. I took a leave of absence from my job to take care of her. In August of 2001, after many doctor visits trying to figure out why her skin had turned so dark and dry, she went to a dermatologist and had a skin biopsy, which came back as scleroderma. I had only known one other person with scleroderma and it scared me. We made an appointment with a rheumatologist and he determined that she did not have scleroderma, but did have dermatomyositis.

During this time, the skin on the back of my hands had become very shiny and a different texture from the rest of the skin. I went to see my dermatologist about the texture of my skin, as well as the hyperpigmentation and hypopigmented skin changes I was experiencing. She took one look at my hands and asked me if I had problems with the cold. When I told her yes, she ordered blood work and suggested I go see my mother's rheumatologist as I probably had a related condition.

She called about two weeks later to tell me my blood work indicated scleroderma but to have it checked by the rheumatologist. The rheumatologist confirmed the diagnosis of diffuse scleroderma on my initial visit to him. Since then, I have had a muscle biopsy, which confirmed polymyositis. I battle flare-ups on what is almost a monthly basis, but it is my faith that keeps me going in spite of it all.

❖❖❖

Marina Paath
Australia

It is February 1, 2004, and here is my story.In May 2001, I noticed unsightly dry skin on my knuckles. I went to my dermatologist who also noticed the bluish color of my fingers. She suspected that I had Raynaud's and sent me for a blood test. The results confirmed that I have scleroderma. I was sent to a rheumatologist who spent an hour and a half checking me while explaining this rare and incurable autoimmune connective tissue disease.

I came home with a pamphlet about the disease and a handful of referrals to undergo pulmonary function tests, CAT scan, echocardiogram (ECG), urine tests for the liver and kidneys, and more blood tests. My head was reeling with the amount of information I had to process and the tests I had to undergo. I had to fit in all these appointments with my teaching schedule at the university and conferences with my divorce lawyers.

Two weeks later I went back to my rheumatologist to find out about the results. My organs functioned well except the lungs, which have minor scarring. My lungs also function below normal for my age, weight and height, but then they never did function normally because I have had mild asthma since 1996 and have to take an inhaler every morning. My rheumatologist referred me to another rheumatologist who specializes in scleroderma.

Dr. Helen Englert has devoted her post-graduate studies to scleroderma research. The number of letters after her name assured me that I am in good hands. My assurance was confirmed when she greeted and ushered me into her office. She is the warmest, most sympathetic, personable, and caring medical specialist I have ever met, and trust me, I have encountered many! She not only diagnosed my physical symptoms but she also approaches my condition holistically. She was pleased to know that I see a psychiatrist for counseling. In addition to the tests I already underwent, she ordered a skin biopsy and performed nail-fold capillaroscopy. The results were nothing to be alarmed about. My condition was diagnosed as mild borderline limited CREST with possible lung involvement.

Psychologically and emotionally I underwent a period of "Why me?" It did not last long because I turned the question into "Why not me?" (Besides, what else can I do?) There is no point in getting angry and fretting. I cannot get rid of it because there is no cure. All I can do, with my doctor's help, is to manage it and accept the fact that life will now be different.

The commencement of 2002 promised a new life as the divorce settlement case concluded. I thought nothing of my new ailment because physically I felt fine; my swollen fingers were just an annoyance. I was mentally and emotionally exhausted and a wreck due to the long, nasty, and phenomenally expensive divorce case. But a new life was not to be. I admitted myself to a private mental clinic for a nervous breakdown and more importantly, to prevent myself from self-harm: I found out that my boyfriend had betrayed me. I simply could not believe that it was happening all over again. I have always held the convictions of not to say 'never again' and that Machiavellian was wrong when he said that "man is basically evil". I guess I was just a trusting, gullible and naive person, not to mention stupid! (All the personality traits I despise and strive hard to avoid, and obviously failed yet again.)

The turning point came when I received a visit from my twenty-one-year-old son. The first thing he said to me when he saw me was, "Why Mum? Can't you cope?" It was the motivation I needed! My own child questioned my coping skills? His super-mum, whom he reluctantly had to model because his own father was too busy with work and social life, was now no longer invincible?

The next day I prepared myself to leave. The first thing on my list was to get spiritual help. Memories of my parents' devotion to religion and those Sunday school classes came flooding back. I contacted a church I visited two years ago for a course. They sent two counselors to see me at the clinic. On Sundays I attended church and on Tuesday evenings I attended Bible study. Spiritually I was developing, as well as forming new friendships, and for the first time in thirty years, I was content with the world.

In June I went to visit some old friends from university in Kuala Lumpur. While there I felt swelling and tightness of my fingers, which I assumed was caused by the heat and humidity. I continued my trip to Singapore and Indonesia, enjoying the freedom and feeling very blessed.

In August I returned to Sydney and began teaching of semester two. I asked my rheumatologist to put me back on prednisone. By September my body was on fire when I attempted to sleep at night. In the morning I felt like I had been hit by a truck. During the day I was in pain and extreme lethargy. I also began to notice that my vision was failing and in class, I would take time delivering my lectures as I had to search for words in order to string sentences together. Some friends began to ask whether I had been sunbathing during my overseas trip because my skin was darker and reddish in color.

I saw Dr. Englert, who quickly organized the tests I had the previous year as well as prescribed many medications. The tests showed that my heart, liver and kidneys were fine, but not my lungs. The CAT scans showed progression of basal interstitial fibrosis. Calcinosis and shininess could be seen around my lower neck. My creatine phosphokinase (CPK) was high, hence the myositis. I was unable to blow dry my hair or lift anything. Thankfully my blood pressure is normal. Dr. Englert suggested intravenous cyclophosphamide instead of methotrexate but I declined because I was terrified of the side effects.

The next six months I had monthly blood tests. In April 2003 I had to inject a much higher dose of methotrexate once a week for five weeks. On the day of the injection and the following day I would feel extremely sick. I could only sprawl on the bed or couch and remain there. Gradually the treatment eased my myositis and lowered the creatine kinase level, but not the lethargy. In the meantime I gained a lot of weight and my facial cheeks were stretched, shiny and chubby. Dr. Englert said that once I get off prednisone, I should get my svelte figure back.

House cleaning that used to take two hours now took the whole day because I had to rest every half hour. I did not have the energy to go out; in fact, I simply could not be bothered. To me, socializing required so much energy and effort. Gone was the vibrant, vivacious party girl and social butterfly.

The worst thing was that I could no longer go to church activities because of the lethargy. I was not confident driving at night because of my poor vision. I found it difficult to focus, and was therefore afraid that my reflexes were slow. For the first time in my teaching career I took a couple of days of sick leave and sprawled on the bed at home. My mild limited CREST had now apparently developed into aggressive systemic diffuse scleroderma.

In early October I was back to a lower dose of oral methotrexate and prednisone. My pulmonary tests showed stabilization, and the creatine kinase level was going down. I responded to treatment! However, in the last weeks of October I suffered from dypsnea (shortness of breath), very dry eyes and mouth, as well as mild gastroesophageal reflux. I wondered if I now have acquired Sjögren's Syndrome.

My lethargy was worse and the swelling and tightness of fingers started again. My lips were thinner, my facial cheeks had hardened, and for the first time in my life, I had cellulite on my legs. When I spoke, my voice quickly became hoarse because of the dryness, and I would have dry coughs. My mouth also felt uncomfortable and tight when I talked.

When I told Dr. Englert that my psychiatrist had prescribed medication for depression, she acknowledged that it is common with chronic illnesses. She then asked me what was happening in the relationship front, to which I answered, "What man in his right mind would take a woman who has a chronic illness?" She held my upper arms, looked me in the eyes and said, "You have a beautiful heart and that is what is important. Your body is not functioning well temporarily and I am trying to help you get a good quality of life." My eyes welled up.

My early positive outlook disappeared because now I physically feel rotten. I am depressed because I can no longer do the things I used to do. I am grieving over the loss of my energy and agility. My lungs would feel like they are on fire when I walk on a slight incline. I have to sit down after I shower, for goodness sake! I feel that I have been cheated by scleroderma.

November saw my faith tested to its limit. An abnormal Pap smear result landed me on the operating table for a cone biopsy. The surgery was fine and the pathology result was not a death sentence, since pre-cancerous cells were identified and treated. So now, on top of all the scleroderma-related tests, I have to have a Pap smear twice a year for the next two years. Attitude-wise I could care less about this latest problem because having scleroderma and its secondary syndromes are shocking enough. Cervical cancer is just another shock to add to the list.

The year 2004 began with an interesting and relaxing holiday traveling around the picturesque north coast of New South Wales with my boyfriend. He talked of marriage and spending the rest of his life with me. I have heard it all before, many times, so my excitement level was pretty neutral. We had numerous and long discussions about fundamental issues in a marriage. Both of us are not young, so between us we have enough baggage to fill a Boeing747 cargo hold. One of the issues, of course, is SD. He is well informed of my condition. I have warned him that one day I may not be able to earn an income and will depend on him financially and physically. I now cannot even perform full-time work. Moreover, my doctor was not keen on me getting pregnant. Age and long-term medication are against me.

At forty-five, I am single. I have three well-adjusted adult children. I am convinced that despite the low quality of life scleroderma gives me, it has brought me closer to my sister, brother, sister-in-law, nephew and nieces, and made me more appreciative of my friendship with Jan and Keith (former work colleagues and bosses as well as beautiful human beings). It has slowed me down so that I can smell the roses.

My faith has given me inner peace, strength and hope. My mother used to say that I am blessed. I agree with her. I have a wonderful eleven-member medical team, family and friends.

Update – February 2004

Yesterday I found the following excerpt in a reply to a sufferer's plea for help on a scleroderma discussion group web site. The sufferer was a twenty-five-year-old woman who had just been diagnosed. She was terrified and in particular worried about not finding a partner, her ability to get pregnant, etc. It reminded me so much of my situation. Recently my boyfriend dumped me primarily because I cannot have children, and I also believe he saw me as a liability, because my earning capacity now is zilch.

Allan is a forty-six-year-old man who was diagnosed with scleroderma in 2001. His reply to her plea strengthens my faith in men; there are genuine ones around. "Lastly, please do not give up hope on finding a mate and having a family. I know that is easy for me to say, since I am married. Believe it or not, there are men in this world who are looking for more than a trophy wife—there are men who look inside rather than outside, men who value and seek out women of intelligence, integrity and compassion. There are men who want a woman with a kind heart and a gentle spirit, not this week's winner of the "hot bod" contest. You do not want a guy who only looks for outer beauty anyway, because outer beauty will ultimately fade, and then what? As with scleroderma, trust in God, the universe or however you think of the higher power to guide you and provide answers."

On my visit to my rheumatologist last week, I told her what happened. She was shocked, upset, said, "It's him, not you," and hugged me. She also said, "You are not good with choosing men, are you?" My doctor is happy with my condition, although quite concerned with the newly apparent Sjögren's. She wanted me to see Professor Dennis Wakefield, an immunologist at Prince of Wales Hospital for management of this secondary syndrome.

Last night, while on a visit to her father, my youngest daughter told my ex-husband of my illness. She had no choice really because she wanted her father to support her financially again this year for her second year of university. She had my approval. I resigned myself to the fact that I should be humble and not be embarrassed of my illness. My daughter told me that her father seemed upset and asked her to give me his regards when he dropped her home. This gesture prompted me to forgive him, a very good move if I want to move on with my life; it is also what I wanted to do all along, to forgive others, a trait which does not come naturally to me.

I hope my story can enlighten other sufferers and caregivers of this awful illness, including how it can affect us psychologically, bearing in mind that it affects sufferers differently and treatments might work for one but not another. One thing that is definite though, you will find comfort, strength and hope in your faith, as I do.

Mary Jane Futrell
North Carolina, USA

I was diagnosed with scleroderma and Raynaud's around December 2002. Before that, I was having trouble with heartburn. My regular doctor tried many different antacids, but none of them worked.

I made an appointment with a gastroenterologist who did an endoscopy around June 2002. That showed inflammation of my stomach, so he referred me to a surgeon, who ordered several more tests.

I had a barium swallow, a pH balance test, and a twenty-four hour pH test. Then finally I had another endoscopy. It showed that my esophagus does not close at all when I swallow. The surgeon suggested that he could do a Nissen Fundoplication. We were not sure if I had scleroderma, but were pretty sure I did, so the doctor said he would do a partial rather than a full wrap, because of the possibility of scleroderma. At this time, I made an appointment with a rheumatologist.

That is when I found out I have scleroderma and Raynaud's. I had the Nissen Fundoplication surgery on February 7, 2003. This surgery made the biggest difference in the world. I have not had heartburn and I can finally sleep at night.

I now sleep with two pillows instead of four. I will need to have another endoscopy done every two years because of the scleroderma.

I am having a lot of joint pain now, and very dry eyes and mouth. My rheumatologist put me medication for the pain and drops for the dry eyes.

It is really hard dealing with this, not knowing how it will affect me. I take it day by day. Nobody really understands unless they are also going through this. Thanks for letting me share this with you!

❖❖❖

Peter Breeze
England, UK

In 1996 I was badly burned by an electrical flashover in a substation and I had to undergo skin grafts to large parts of my body. After twelve months I was well enough to return to work, though not in the job I had been doing. My life gradually got back to normal until I noticed my right elbow was getting very stiff. I went back to see the plastic surgeon who had done my skin grafts and various treatments were tried. These included emollients and intensive physical therapy, all to no avail.

After these treatments failed it was decided that an operation would have to be performed to release the ever-stiffening elbow. I got as far as the operating theater and was given a general anesthetic. When I awoke the surgeon told me he had changed his mind and had not done the operation and further tests would have to be done. I had a biopsy done which proved inconclusive and the surgeon seemed baffled.

Eventually my other elbow stiffened up and my fingers became swollen and stiff. Many months went by and the doctors seemed completely bemused by my condition. Eventually the skin of my legs became hard and shiny and I was having increasing trouble walking. Also by this time my left hand had contracted so much that I had to wear a protective piece of plastic on my palm to prevent my fingernails growing through the skin. At this point I underwent another biopsy, this time with skin from my legs. The results confirmed I had scleroderma. I also have Raynaud's along with that.

Although it is not nice to be told you have an incurable condition, I was relieved just to know they had at last found out what was wrong with me. My case was handed over to a rheumatologist and I was treated with several medications. My condition has greatly improved; my legs are almost normal and some of the movement has returned to my hands. Although I cannot work at the moment, my life is getting back to normal and I am starting to enjoy myself again.

I think the hardest part of this for me was not knowing what was wrong with me, and I hope that for the sake of others that diagnostic techniques improve in the future. The strange thing about all this is that the areas where I had skin grafts did not go hard like the surrounding skin, and remained soft and supple.

In conclusion, I would like to tell fellow sufferers not to be afraid, and to ask for help. All my friends and family helped me in my worst times and they help me maintain the positive attitude that I still have today.

Steve Dickson
England, UK

I am forty-two, married with a son, and live in England. My symptoms started in 1993, when I noticed my fingers became cold even though it was summer and the temperatures were mild.

This started about one year after my dad died of a sudden heart attack. The next thing I knew, the little finger on my right hand started to curl inwards. This is when I had my first test in a hospital, which was a skin biopsy taken from my forearm. From this my rheumatologist confirmed I had secondary Raynaud's with diffuse scleroderma. He told me not to worry unduly, but to find out as much as I could from leaflets about how to ease the symptoms.

Before long, more of my fingers were curling up and making my life harder, especially since I had a manual job in the aerospace industry. Five years later, after having tried my best to put up with the pain in my fingers and wrists, I asked to be moved into a more comfortable role at work. To their credit, they could not do enough for me. I have an assessor who visits me at my workstation to see if there are more things they can do to help me work at a computer. Even though I type slower than other people, I can draw on my experience of working on machinery to maintain a rewarding job.

In 1998, I had a MRI which showed I have lung involvement. My lungs are currently eighty percent efficient, and seem to be holding steady. I went on a treatment of intravenous drugs to try to combat the fibrosis, but it did not seem to work.

During the last five years, my condition has slowly deteriorated, but I am still hanging in there working, and I still manage to drive. In England we have the National Health Service, which allows us to have treatment in hospitals, so we do not have to worry about paying for that treatment. But this illness has definitely curtailed my earning power. My wife also struggles to maintain a full time job, whilst having to do my share of the chores at home. She has had to settle for temporary work, so that she can be more flexible.

All this does come at a cost, especially when I had to purchase a newer car with automatic transmission, and all the other gadgets that aid driving. My house needs adapting also to allow me to shower safely, and I have just been assessed for and been given a wheelchair because my right ankle is painful when I walk. I will use the wheelchair to go shopping or on other outings.

I am trying to claim benefits, but I have found that because this disease is rare, it seems more difficult than if I had something everyone knows about, such as arthritis. But I am sure I will get the benefits eventually!

Thank you for reading my story; it helps to share thoughts. I would gladly welcome hearing from you, especially from male patients, as there are so very few of us.

I send the warmest thoughts to all of you in 'our community'.

Amy Barr
Ohio, USA

I am thirty-eight, a mother of three children, a wife and a full time pharmacist in a pediatric hospital. In February and March of this year, I became very intolerable of the cold. I live in the Northeast and it is not easy to get out of the cold here!

Within a few weeks of noticing how cold I always was, I started hurting all over, as if I had the flu. The fatigue, the muscle weakness and especially the shortness of breath whenever I tried to do anything remotely physical never got better, but only worse. It got to the point where I could not even lift a laundry basket of clothes and walk downstairs to our laundry room. My upper arms and shoulders ached when I would wash my hair in the shower.

I had seen my physician three times, and had gotten a tentative diagnosis of fibromyalgia. At the third appointment (when I was getting fed up with how I felt) I was told I seemed a bit "nervous." Um, yeah. My body was falling apart around me, I cannot do the simple things with my children that just a few months ago I could, and no one had a reason for it.

He referred me to a rheumatologist, and I had to wait almost four months for an appointment. While waiting, I ended up hospitalized for four days right before Memorial Day. It was very hard for me to breathe, and I could not even walk up a flight of stairs at work without sweating and breathing very heavy. I got the million dollar cardiac work up that noted "mild restrictive" lung disease, but no one followed up any further, since I did not smoke. I left with an inhaler and was told to maybe try to exercise a bit more.

My appointment finally came with the rheumatologist. He took one look at my edematous (swollen) hands and thick fingers and said he was going to do a full work up for lupus. He did not know what was going on, but he was sure it was some sort of connective tissue disease.

One month later at my follow-up appointment on October 10, 2003, I was told I have limited systemic sclerosis with the CREST syndrome variant. My antinuclear antibodies (ANA) were high, and I had a very high anticentromere antibody (ACA) titer. After I let it sink in over the weekend, I called the pulmonologist that read my pulmonary function test (PFT) reports when I was hospitalized in May and asked him to go over them again, now knowing that I have scleroderma. He called back and scheduled me for a follow-up pulmonary function test (PFT) and a chest X ray. He asked me how in the world I knew to follow up on this. I told him I had done some reading. He was quite impressed. I have since done a lot more reading, and have joined a support group. I am getting copies of all of my lab work and tests, and keeping them in my 'derma file'.

My family feels that I may be in denial about this disease. I feel more relieved to know that this has not been all in my head these last nine months.

Although I am not happy about what is to come in my life, I am happy that I know what it is I am fighting against. I know now why it is that I do not have a bowel movement for four or five days, then have diarrhea for two days! I know now why it hurts to walk after I have been sitting for an hour or two. I know why my hands swell and ache and I know what these funky little red lines are on my chest and neck. I know why food gets stuck in my throat every once in a while, or why I cannot drink liquids very fast sometimes. I also know now why my bowling average has dropped like a rock...wish I could fix that!

Betty Fults
Tennessee, USA

Hi, my name is Betty. I have CREST scleroderma. It took two years for them to find out what I have. I went through two surgeries on my colon for nothing and I have gone downhill ever since.

My skin is not too bad. I have a little tightness on my fingers with the shiny stuff (sclerodactyly). My main problem is in my organs. The scleroderma has badly affected my stomach. The doctors say it does not work anymore. I have a feeding tube and a drainage tube. I got to where I am because I was throwing up everyday and I lost a lot of weight. My weight was two hundred and fourteen pounds before I became ill, which came on quickly, and then I went down to one hundred and twenty-four pounds. That is when I got all the tubes. I can still eat but the food just sits in my stomach and then the bile overflows, which was why I was throwing up all the time.

It has been a horrible experience for me and my family. I feel like just pulling the tubes out and forget it all. I cry all the time, stay depressed, and worry every minute of every day.

I would like to talk with someone who has the tubes also. Maybe that will help me.

Most days I get up sick and for the past year I have to sleep sitting straight up in a chair. I cannot lay down flat and this is really getting to me. I do not know how much more I can take.

◆❖◆

Beverly Hutton Block
New York, USA

I was born with a cleft palate and a nasal voice. I had two operations, but they were not successful. I still have a nasal voice but talk a little bit better now.

When my mom fed me as a baby the milk/formula kept running out of my mouth so it took a long time to feed me. They did not know anything about cleft palate back in the early 1950s. Now children can get operations for it, so they don't have to go through life being tortured and teased by other children. I was a misfit and felt like I did not belong. I never had any friends and I came home crying daily from school.

In ninth grade I was pulled out of public school and put into private school. While there I was pretty much left alone. I graduated number thirty-two out of thirty-three girls in 1971, but at least I graduated, and now I am an honor student and I plan to finish by bachelor's degree online.

Now I am fifty-one years old and I began experiencing symptoms of asthma and Raynaud's disease around 1996.

I was going to college, before online courses and degrees were available, and was noticing shortness of breath while going up and down three flights of stairs to my classroom twice daily. I noticed that my fingers and toes were getting colder, turning white, then blue, and finally turning numb, especially when I got cold. I would go into the college bathroom and rub my fingers under warm water (not hot, as I did not want to burn myself.)

From then on, I started getting worse, and on top of it all, I was going through menopause at the same time. I graduated with an Associate Degree in Business, and then I started getting worse. I was overtired and needed naps in the afternoon, and as pain was slowly getting the better of me, I finally went to the doctor.

After a physical exam and blood work, he told me I had Raynaud's and the CREST variation of systemic scleroderma, skin tightening on my fingers (sclerodactyly), along with fibromyalgia and chronic fatigue syndrome (CFS). I had already had gastric reflux and a hiatal hernia, both of which were giving me trouble with swallowing and causing me to throw up food as soon as I ate it. I also get frequent stomach ulcers. Whenever I get colds or sinus infections, my asthma seems to get worse. What a mouthful of diseases for one person to handle all at once!

The doctor put me on a pain reliever and medication for my stomach ulcers. Once the ulcers healed, I was able to eat normally. However, I still occasionally get episodes of vomiting, and then I get put back on the ulcer medication. Now it is available over-the-counter and is less expensive.

Meanwhile, I wanted to go on for my bachelor's degree but could not go to college. I was bitterly disappointed, but a year later I got my first computer and was able to continue my education online.

In March 1999, a year after my mom died (my dad had passed away seven years earlier), I met my new boyfriend online, as well.

We got married on February 2, 2000, Ground Hog Day. We both waited for love and married late in life. My husband has multiple sclerosis (MS), and is no longer in remission. He is going through some pretty tough symptoms. We are both on Social Security disability, so we are still poor, barely able to pay the rent and our bills. We hold many stoop sales (garage sales), just to be able to put food on the table.

Several years later I was diagnosed with rheumatoid arthritis, osteoarthritis, and high blood pressure. Just this year, I was also diagnosed with diabetes.

I never had any children, and now that I am through menopause, I cannot have any, so we are childless. Luckily, we have each other, and that is all that matters!

Boo
Vermont, USA

I was born in 1961. I am a college graduate. I was always hard working and very active socially. I live hard and I play hard.

In late 1992, I caught a virus that manifested as a flu-like illness with a bright red pinpoint rash covering my legs. Three months later I was hospitalized due to dehydration after the prolonged flu-like illness.

About six months after that, my arms were numb, sore, and swollen. The swelling was so bad that the nerves in my arms were malfunctioning and the pain became unbearable at night. I was diagnosed with carpal tunnel syndrome and had a surgical release done on my right wrist. This did help tremendously in the short term.

After the surgery I was referred to a rheumatologist. The surgeon said, "You have what appears to be full-blown rheumatoid arthritis (RA)." After consulting with the specialist and seeking a second, confirming opinion, I began treatment at the local university's rheumatology clinic.

Due to the fatigue and general ill health I was experiencing, I left work and did not return for two and a half years. The road to becoming diagnosed was long!

The rheumatologist knew I had a problem but was unwilling to put a label on it for some time. My symptoms, at times, pointed toward multiple sclerosis (MS). Finally in 1994, it was labeled as CREST syndrome, which is a form of systemic scleroderma. I have been treated with several medications, cortisone injections, various anti-inflammatories, and kindness.

Ten years later, I am having blood work drawn annually and am seeing my specialist for a progress report every six months. I also have X rays taken every eighteen months to monitor the calcification problems.

I have been back to work full-time for five years, and continue on a maintenance dose of anti-inflammatories to help control the pain. The fatigue continues to be a constant battle. At forty-one, I feel old!

I have particular difficulty with my hips, hands, wrists and spine. I have noticed increasing problems with my vision with floaters, and I have tremendous disfigurement around my hips. In certain areas I am completely void of muscle mass and strength, or the connective tissues remain hardened, rendering them useless. My skin has lost most of its elasticity and I am slow to heal.

I continue with low-impact exercise and hope to always push forward with my life. The worst part of the experience has been that I can never get complete relief, which is physically and mentally exhausting. As a result, I have been quite depressed at times. The good news is that the progression of the sclerosis is no longer apparent. In fact, even though I have residual damage, it appears that it may have been knocked out by one of my medications or possibly it burned itself out over time.

What a crazy disease! The uncertainty of the prognosis is completely frustrating. I have good and bad days. I may retire to a warmer climate, but I would hate to lose out on the wonderful New England change of seasons.

Carol Farley
Indiana, USA

For the last two years my hands and feet have been going numb. At first I did not think much of it since I had three herniated discs and thought it could have been from that. I told my doctor about the numbness and he did not say anything about it. The last two winters were really tough for me. I could not tolerate the cold. My hands and feet would go completely white, and I would shake all over.

One day I woke up and I could barely move. I never hurt so badly in my life! Walking even bothered me. I kept thinking to myself that I am only thirty-three years old, and that this is not something I can just blow off. For two weeks it was awful! The pain all over my body woke me up in the night. I decided to quit being stubborn and to see my family doctor. I told him about the pain I was in and I also told him about my hands and feet and how I could not tolerate the cold anymore. He decided to run some blood work.

I knew when I got a call at home from him that it was not good. He told me that my antinuclear antibodies (ANA) were extremely high and he wanted me to see a rheumatologist. So I was thinking that maybe I had a mild case of arthritis. Others told me that it was probably a mistake that the lab had made. I knew it was not a mistake because of the way I was feeling.

When I went to see this specialist, I was really nervous because there were three doctors examining me, asking a lot of questions, and talking about all different kinds of diseases it could be. Needless to say, I was scared!

Once again I was asked to have more blood tests. I got another phone call at home and was asked to come in the next morning to discuss my results. I was told that I had a very rare disease called CREST with scleroderma. I had no clue what was involved with this diagnosis, so I could not ask the right questions. They just told me I would be on medication and that I had to get blood work every three months.

I have done a lot of researching since last week and now I am really confused. I have found the International Scleroderma Network web site to be the most helpful! I am afraid of not knowing what my future holds. I feel so alone right now and it would be nice to talk with someone who understands what I am going through.

◆ ❖ ◆

Carrie Hernandez
Florida, USA

All this started in 1995, as far as receiving any diagnosis. First, I was diagnosed with breast cancer. I went through radiation and chemotherapy.

Then I went to a rheumatologist. He first diagnosed me with fibromyalgia. I had swim therapy and that helped some. Then he left the area. I was still having extreme discomfort so I went to a new rheumatologist who had replaced my first one. She did blood work and my antinuclear antibodies (ANA) test result was very high. That is when she told me I had CREST scleroderma. The last ANA test showed it had elevated substantially. After much research, I was rather concerned, especially when I found out there was no cure.

I have learned to live with most of the pain. But I find that when I become very upset, or catch a cold, or have an allergy attack, the condition worsens.

Then my husband was injured in 1996, and the accident left him a quadriplegic. He was having a lot of pain that was incapacitating. I am his sole caregiver as well as my own.

I have no support within the community. It seems that caregivers of quadriplegics go into some kind of hiding. Therefore, we are left with no support and with no support for my illness.

I am also under the care of a psychiatrist who just keeps shaking his head at how well I have maintained my life. He has offered me a bed at the Pavilion, an inpatient hospital facility, if I ever need it.

Right now I am trying to deal with issues at home and also issues pertaining to my father's death in January.

It seems that it never ends. I have a key chain that says "I cannot have a crisis, my schedule is full." But it always seems there is one crisis after another.

Update – July 2004

I am having more problems with Raynaud's. I am also beginning to have chest tightening and irregular heart beats. I have been going through a new series of testing to see where I am at now. Even though I normally have low blood pressure, it has now dropped to the 80's/over 50's. My doctor says that I have to stay hydrated. That is not a problem as this disease also affects my thirst. The only thing that takes care of the thirst is drinking six to ten glasses of water a day.

I will also be having nerve conduction studies done to see if carpal tunnel is causing my arms and hands to go to sleep no matter what I do. Sometimes they are so bad I will not drive as I do not trust myself to handle the car in a tight situation. The numbness has also affected my legs. I find if I sit too long in one position my legs go to sleep and then it takes a lot of effort for me to get up.

My husband passed away on December 23, 2003, two days before Christmas. This first year so far has been the hardest. I thought I had prepared myself for the inevitable, but I find that I really did not. I miss John terribly.

I had to move from our house because the memories were really sending me into a deep depression. I am doing better in that regard, but the pain and the loss are still very much in the forefront. The only comfort I can take is that John is in a better place and not a prisoner of a body that did not work. When he passed it had been exactly seven years from the day I took him home. Everyone said I would not be taking him home at that time. Like I said at the services, I had him to love for all those seven years.

Danielle LeBlanc
Canada

I would love to share my story of CREST scleroderma that I have been living with for over six years now.

When I was young I was sick a lot. My mom brought me to see the doctor frequently. All he had to say was "growing pains" because I was young. I would feel sick mostly in the morning and after a few hours would feel better. My parents always thought of it as an excuse to miss school. It all started with my hands. They would be swollen and turn white and blue in cold weather.

As years went on I kept feeling worse and worse. Finally I went to see my doctor again for more tests. It was in 1998 that I was diagnosed with CREST scleroderma. When my doctor gave me the news I told him thank you! He was amazed by that response. I then said, "Well, at least now I know I am not losing my mind."

My family understood as little about this illness as I did. All I understood at first is that it was like arthritis. Little did I know it was much more serious than that.

I was able to finish school with no problems and went to college. I even worked tough jobs with no problems. As years went on, I was amazed at how it progressed. I was diagnosed with Sjögren's syndrome a year after being diagnosed with CREST. The pain was unbearable at times. I would start to miss more and more work. Then I got diagnosed with fibromyalgia. At first I thought it was just a way for the doctor to tell me I had pain. I took it as an excuse and thought he did not know what else to tell me. I came to find out it is a very serious illness as well.

In November 2002, I stopped working. I figured if I wanted a halfway decent life that it would be the best thing for me. That was the hardest part. I am hoping one day that I will be able to return to work.

The disease continues to progress as I was diagnosed with acid reflux in early 2004.

I have a lot of support from my fiancé and also my family and friends. I do have better days than others, but the support I get from everyone around me helps me get through a lot. Their support helps me realize that I am not necessarily living with this illness alone.

❖❖❖

Dawna
Utah, USA

I have rarely heard the term CREST and am interested to learn more from real people about this disease.

I am in my mid-forties and was diagnosed with Raynaud's when I was about twenty-two. The doctor also said that I have fibromyalgia that in my experience is a wastebasket term for 'we do not really know what you have nor do we care.'

I have had antinuclear antibodies (ANA) ranging from 1:80 to 1:320. My symptoms range from very painful hands when they are cold to burning hot when they are warm. The bones are recently beginning to become quite painful at times. My skin seems to get tight over my knuckles and turns white when I grasp things or put my hand into a fist. I have esophageal spasms, motility problems, and severe acid reflux with pyloric stenosis. As of yet, I have no real problems swallowing or chest pain even when I take my prescription medicine for reflux.

I have severe tinnitus in both ears and have had temporomandibular joint (TMJ) surgery on both sides of my face, which was mostly due to the impact of an auto airbag injury. I also have irritable bowel syndrome (IBS) and sciatica, as well as neck, back and hip pain. I have skin sensitivity to hot and cold, some fabrics, and even touch at times. I frequently get itchy rashes on my arms legs, stomach, back, and hips; as well as paresthesia (a fuzzy numb feeling) on arms, hands and face.

Could this be CREST with an overlap of something else? I had a friend tell me she thought it sounds like lupus. My doctor does not seem to think so.

Most of the time, I am tired and hurting. I am also tired of going to doctors. I was in a car accident two and a half years ago and have had four surgeries since then, three surgeries on my right hand, as well as the bilateral TMJ surgery.

I feel as if I have used my life's ration of fuel and that I am existing on fumes.

❖❖❖

Donna Murray
Vermont, USA

It all started with an infection at the end of my index finger in December 1999. My finger became red, inflamed and sore to touch. After a few weeks I went to my doctor and he said there was an infection and there was no way for it to come out. He cut a hole through my finger and placed a wick in it to take out the infection. I think I would have rather kept the infection as it was a very painful procedure.

Then he sent me to another doctor who did blood work and sent me home still not knowing what was going on. When the results came back he suggested that I see a rheumatologist, which I did. The rheumatologist said I had an autoimmune disease, or what is known as CREST scleroderma. He also said that I had Raynaud's. That was in February 2000.

I get ulcers on the tips of my fingers, my skin is tight on my hands and the skin often cracks open under my fingernails. This is quite painful. All this doctor has done is put me on blood pressure medication, to help keep my kidneys from failing, and run certain tests to make sure my lungs and my heart are still working okay.

I get the purple fingers and the pain when it is cold outside, and I am always wearing gloves. I live in the Northeast and we have cold winters and they are tough to get through.

It is very hard to even make a fist as my skin on my hands is tight. I have trouble with my skin being very dry all the time and I think I have tried every lotion on the market.

I am not sure where this disease will take me or how long before other things start happening. I just try to take it day by day. Some are better than others and every morning when I wake up, I know that I still have a chance.

◆ ❖ ◆

Jerri Sue DeTray
Ohio, USA

I am a thirty-eight-year-old mom. I was twenty-one when I first noticed that my fingers, toes and lips were turning colors. It scared me. My sister was going to medical school, so I went over to her house and grabbed her medical book. I finally found something that was just like my symptoms. It was Raynaud's.

I showed my sister and she told me that I should notify my doctor. My doctor sent me to the hospital for some tests, which confirmed I had Raynaud's. Then Dr. Roode wanted me to see a rheumatologist named Dr. Harmon. She told me that I could eventually have lupus or scleroderma. I just thought she must be kidding. Her words went in one ear and out the other.

It was not until my diagnosis of scleroderma that I knew I was in for a long haul. My mom said that she had thought it was their fault for my having this. She remarked that our blood did not match, and that from the day I was born I have had health problems. I was allergic to everything, even water. My doctor was worried but said I should be getting some nutrients, because the water would stay down for awhile before it would come back up. Finally, I outgrew that allergy.

Growing up I can remember being really tired all the time. I would go to school and then come home and take a nap. My mom told the doctor what was going on. He simply told her I must need the extra sleep and not to worry. I always seemed to catch colds a lot. I had pneumonia a few times and always had sore throats.

One time in junior high school I had gotten out of bed and could not walk. The doctor could not explain why. He thought maybe I had hit my knee on something, as I was a teenage girl who loved to run and climb trees, anything an active teenager would do. Eventually, the pain in my right leg went away. Then one day my right knee started giving me problems. I could not join the track team because of it. It was so painful, but that also went away.

I had my children at the young age of seventeen. My parents could not believe that I wanted to try and have children knowing I would be too tired to take care of them. But I fooled everyone. I thought I was in love and wanted to get married and have children. I have three children. All my children were born prematurely. My oldest son, Michael, weighed three pounds and five ounces and is now twenty-one years old. Joshua weighed four pounds and five ounces and is now nineteen, and Andrea weighed in at four pounds and seven and a half ounces and is presently eighteen years old. They all deny that anything is wrong with me and get scared when something does go wrong. I am the only parent my children have, as their father committed suicide at a young age. I was not married to him at that time.

Over the years nothing seemed to really go wrong until 1992 when I started to have pain in my knees again. I went to a doctor in California after I had remarried and moved there. The doctor ran some tests and thought I had a connective tissue disorder. He gave me medication for Raynaud's. I felt a little better.

We moved back to Ohio in 1994 and I started having problems with my right knee again. I had developed calcium deposits and they oozed nasty white stuff for a few weeks and then cleared up. The infections in my knee happened on and off for years and did not clear up until 2002. I also started having reflux and had to see a gastroenterologist and have an endoscopy. I was told I had Barrett's disease, and given medicine for that.

I had enough of all this, so I quit going to the doctor, except for my family doctor. After I started having more problems with my right knee in 1996, I was told I had scleroderma and I chose not to see that rheumatologist ever again. I was in denial. During that year the movie "For Hope" came out. I watched that movie and was terrified by it.

I called my second husband who was in the military (USMC) and told him that I had been diagnosed with scleroderma. I tried to explain what it was. Two weeks after that he came home and asked me for a divorce. That is when I went into a severe depression. I was losing someone I loved very much and thought was my soul mate. He told me it was not me or my children, but that it was him. Later I found out there was another woman involved.

I met my third husband through my children and his. We dated for six years and got married on October 25, 2002. Then my health problems started in again. I had knee surgery in February 2003. They removed the calcium deposits because it would not heal. I was taking a lot of antibiotics, and started having problems with my bowels. I now have ulcerative colitis, a hiatal hernia, high blood pressure, and thyroid problems.

Life is so grand right now! I had a lot of problems with the bowels and we thought it was diverticulitis at first. I spent a lot of time in the hospital during February through April 2003. I was in the hospital for my thirty-eighth birthday, which was not what I wanted.

Finally, they did a colonoscopy after my second hospitalization for bleeding and diarrhea. They told me I had ulcerative colitis. I was so scared and thought I was going to have colon cancer, but I do not. Then I had to have another scope down my esophagus. The Barrett's was no longer there, but they told me that I have a hiatal hernia, and I cannot have surgery for the hernia, due to the colitis.

I had a lung test in April 2003 and found my lungs have started to harden. I am on an inhaler and I do not think it is helping. My chest feels heavy. I feel very tired and run down every day, and my right hand and foot are also bothering me.

I wish I could twinkle my nose and this would be gone. My nickname is Sam (which is why I say I wish I could twinkle my nose.)

Johnny Barkett
Alabama, USA

I am a thirty-nine-year-old white male and single father of a brilliant ten-year-old boy. Once upon a time I was also a Wireless Telecom engineer and a Gulf War Vet.

The onset was in 1995. As of 2003, I have just won the fight to save my left foot. I spent the previous year and half fighting to save my big toe, but it had to go, because the pain was so unbearable. The infection had moved into my foot. After repeated surgeries to clean the debris and the wound area where my big toe used to be, it finally came down to the surgery. Finally, Dr. Fred Meyer, Professor of Orthopedics at the University of South Alabama Hospital, and his team managed a successful skin graft.

I found that quality of life soon becomes very important in decision-making, when there is so much immobility and pain. Since 1995, I have also lost most of my fingertips. Early on, before they diagnosed scleroderma, which took four years, the gastroesophageal reflux disease (GERD) had caused so much scar tissue that I had to have laser surgery on my windpipe to widen it back to normal.

On a daily basis I still fight the pain from rheumatoid arthritis, stomach upset and irritable bowel. It is difficult just doing daily living tasks like dressing, brushing teeth, folding clothes, or walking without all the tools God gave me to start with. Then there is the occasional depression and psychological symptoms of how this really affects my life and relationships.

Then, add on the physical aspects of learning to live with pain and deal with the side effects of the drugs. And let us not forget the financial burden with trying to live on fifty percent of salary for six months, if we are lucky to have a disability plan at work. And also learning how Social Security pays out, fighting with disability insurance plans and having to renew it every two years, as if my 'stuff' is going to grow back!

I am blessed to have been given the mental capacity to deal with these challenges. I am sure many others give up, and as we know, stress is a large contributing factor to the cycle of this disease.

My first symptoms started in 1995 after I moved to a colder climate from living fifteen years in a warm one. My left middle index finger seemed to have developed a nail fungus-type infection. It would heal, then the infection would come back for several months. Finally, it got worse and I could tell it was not healing. The doctors really did not have a clue about scleroderma at that time. They only mentioned that I had Raynaud's. They ran test after test and still nothing. I finally lost my finger halfway down because they were really uncertain as to what the problem was.

"Quit fixing the symptoms," I said, "and fix the problem!" My finger was dead so they finally chopped it off. Since that first onset, most of my problems came from injuries that would heal in a matter of days for most people but did not heal for me.

I now live in the 'deep south' for the warm climate. However, I still have problems, but not near as bad as when I lived in the colder area. I have a huge family, but nobody else in my family has anything like this disease.

Using my own research process I scanned the Internet. To my intrigue I found that CREST is well documented and that scleroderma is often triggered by environmental exposures to toxins, but nobody will back it up. When I looked at this list it all became clear for me.

When I was in the Navy, for seven years I used solvents to clean the electronics equipment on jets. Many of those chemicals are now listed as the "Super Fund Top Twenty Toxins." The main one I used that had no prescribed safety precautions was trichloroflouroethylene, which is basically Freon® in a spray can. The more research I did, the more positive I became that this was my 'scleroderma trigger'.

Much of the information is above my head, but as an engineer I am pretty well-educated and know how to add one plus one equals two; too bad the Veterans Administration (VA) does not use the same math. I have been battling with them for three years.

I have learned we should not let the health care system run us. We are paying the bill, so we should make sure we get what we want and deserve. If we do not see eye to eye with our doctor, we should get another doctor! We can also call our congressman and senators. They have special liaisons on staff to help get our benefits in order.

We learn who our friends are very quickly when we are ill. If we have tried to move along in relationships and run into brick walls, it is probably not our fault. Sometimes it is a shame how vanity and money often matter more to our significant others. No wonder the divorce rate is fifty percent and climbing. If we are not like "Ken and Barbie" we might as well swim up the creek without the paddle. There should be a singles dating service for those of us with this disease!

◆❖◆

Joy M. Warren
Washington, USA

I had heard that the forties are the best years of life. Well, on July 3, 2002, two months after my fortieth birthday, I was diagnosed with CREST scleroderma with Raynaud's. What a fun day!

I have been married to a wonderful man for seventeen years and we have two precious daughters ages fifteen and thirteen, those wonderful teenage years, but actually they are pretty good kids. I also have been a hairstylist for twenty-two years, the last two as my own boss.

I have had Raynaud's since I was about twenty-three, with no other problems with my hands. As time went by, my family doctor noticed my hands were starting to swell. About twelve years ago he sent me to a rheumatologist who mumbled something about possibly having some sort of connective tissue disease. He did not seem too worried.

So every year my doctor would check my hands, and every year he noticed my Raynaud's was worse. About four or five years ago he ran some blood work for antinuclear antibodies (ANA), which showed that a connective tissue disease was active.

Every year my hands would look a little worse, and then red spots started to appear on my face. I thought they were from aging. My doctor always asked me if I had difficulty swallowing. I told him I didn't, that I just had a lot of heartburn and used a lot of antacids. Last May he decided that I needed to see a specialist again. Thank goodness it was not the same one!

My first appointment with the rheumatologist was three hours long. They examined me from head to toe, and based on my symptoms they knew what I had. I am on a calcium channel blocker for Raynaud's, a proton pump inhibitor for heartburn, and an anti-platelet agent for the Raynaud's. My pulmonary function test (PFT) results were a little low.

Living is day by day. I try not to complain. My hands ache quite a bit. It is kind of scary not knowing when or what will turn up next. It is like having a time bomb waiting to go off. I tease my doctors by telling them that my bathroom is starting to look like a mini-pharmacy.

I just know that I have to let go and not try to control everything around me. I am learning and trying the hard way but I will get there. In the meantime, I am very thankful for the good days!

◆ ❖ ◆

Lynn Francis
England, UK

When I was very young my grandmother always said, "Cold hands, warm heart." Bless her.

At the age of fifty in July 2001, in the middle of a mini heat wave, my hands were freezing and I finally accepted that this was not normal. I had to tell my doctor that my hands were cold. Can you imagine how stupid I felt? But I did not have to worry because my doctor was, and still is, the best. He immediately suspected Raynaud's and started me on medication for it. Great! Sorted! Problem solved!

On August 13, 2001, I had an infection on my right middle finger. My doctor phoned our local hospital, and I had to go there straight away. I had to have my wedding ring cut off. I was sent for blood tests and X rays and told I would probably have to stay overnight as they suspected osteomyelitis, but I had to wait for the surgeon to confirm. He said there was nothing wrong and told me to go home and take aspirin.

Six days later, I was in so much pain my husband took me to the hospital and they told me there was no connection to Raynaud's. I went on holiday from August 27th to September 11th, but I was in constant pain. On September 16th, my husband, Jim, could not stand it anymore either. I went back to the hospital where, at last, I was taken seriously. Part of my finger was removed as it was too far gone to save.

When my doctor heard about this he told me I would probably lose more of my finger and he was going to send letters to all concerned, and "kick arses" (his words, not mine). He was the one who told me about The Raynaud's Association.

By the beginning of October, I was under the care of another doctor in the Connective Tissue and Rheumatology Department who confirmed Raynaud's and scleroderma. He also told me that my medication for Raynaud's had to be gradually increased, and he prescribed medications for heartburn and pain. When I went home and reflected on the past three months, I just could not take it all in. It felt like it must be happening to someone else.

"Hey, I am just ordinary," I thought. Well, on the 17th of September I saw a "fingers and hands" expert. I think she probably saved my life if not my sanity. She said I would have to have more of that finger taken off. I was not happy about it, but at least I was not frightened anymore.

So on November 11th my finger was amputated just above the top knuckle. Unfortunately an infection set in. I was put on antibiotics, along with all the other drugs, which meant I was on twenty-three pills per day. My husband Jim said, "That is nearly one per hour."

Never mind, we are getting there, or so we thought. Wrong! On December 1st, I was back at the hospital with a worse infection! I was given three bags of antibiotics on a drip, and more capsules.

The doctor said, "If there is no improvement...". Well, there was no improvement. Can you guess the next bit? I have left out some of the stuff, but I have got it all in a diary if anyone wants to know about it.

On February 1, 2002, I went into the hospital to have an Iloprost infusion by a syringe pump. I had to stay for five days as that is how long the treatment takes. Whilst I was in the hospital I met, for the first time, a fellow sufferer. It broke my heart. She was far worse than me. All I could do was offer support and understanding. How humble I felt.

On February 28, 2002, I had some more of my finger taken off.

With all that has happened to me, and is still happening, here I am. As you all know, it is never over, but at least I can close that particular chapter and be ready for the next, which I am not looking forward to. But with the help of my family and friends and the wonderful medical team, rare though they are, I know I can make it.

On October 3, 2001, I was a volunteer patient for the Royal College of Surgeons examinations held at Orsett Hospital, because I was, at the time, quite a rare case. I was treated like a queen. I received a thank-you letter afterwards saying that forty-seven of the sixty-five students passed the exam, which equates to seventy percent of the candidates making the grade.

I send my warmest love to sufferers and treaters.

◆ ❖ ◆

Mark Burnett
Canada

My name is Mark Burnett, and I was diagnosed with Raynaud's about fourteen years ago. It began when I started to get extremely painful fingers and feet while playing hockey, so I went to see a local dermatologist. He diagnosed me with Raynaud's and explained that it was very important for me to quit playing hockey to prevent it from getting worse. That was very difficult for me, since I had played hockey for over fifteen years.

I was put on some medication and given a very strict diet to follow. After using the medicine and dieting for over a year, the Raynaud's was under very good control. Then I decided to stop my medication and the diet and I did not return to the doctor. I was very frustrated and maybe this was not the best idea, but being stubborn, it was a choice I had decided to make.

Over the next few years I began playing hockey again, even though it was very painful, and I mean painful! I also started working at a job that required working outdoors in -30° Celsius weather all day every day, working with vibrating equipment most of the time.

After a few years I could not do this anymore, so I quit hockey again and I went back to school to become a graphic designer/illustrator. After graduating near the top of my class, I found it difficult to obtain work for various reasons, including the fact that I cannot use my hands for long periods of time without them cramping up. Therefore, I decided to open my own small graphics business, which allows me to work and stretch out the hours at various times, which I could not do at a nine-to-five job. So far the going is slow, but who knows what the future holds!

Recently, after having problems with my flexibility and more digital ulcers and also ulcers on my elbows, I went back to see my doctor. A new specialist diagnosed me with CREST scleroderma. Initially the diagnosis was not a big deal to me, but after recently having a daughter I decided that it may be a good idea to look into the problem a bit more. The information I found has not eased my mind. There are many good stories, but also some really nasty ones. I have not read many stories about males with the problem, so I decided to write mine.

I am going to Toronto to see another specialist in a month to hopefully get more answers. Wishing everyone health and happiness!

◆ ❖ ◆

Marthie Duminey
South Africa

My name is Marthie and I live in a small town that developed around a chemical and petrochemical industry in this area in South Africa. The town itself is close to a big river, the Vaalriver, and in summer is quite lush and green, although winter finds everything quite grey as we get a lot of frost here.

I have been a single parent for ten years and have three children: a son who is twenty-seven; a daughter who is twenty-three; and a son who is fifteen.

After the birth of my daughter, I started feeling tired. I went to several doctors and had lots of tests done. In the end all that I achieved was that they probably thought I was a hypochondriac. Thereafter I just let matters be. This lasted eighteen years.

Then after potting some plants at work, my hands started itching like mad. My hands turned blue and then white. Not knowing what it was, I joked about it! The itching nearly drove me insane and the doctor prescribed cortisone, which I did not like to take but had no option as the itching was really bad. I was referred to a dermatologist, who prescribed cortisone and many different soaps and creams. This was very costly with no positive results.

I was busy studying for my national diploma in safety. Trying to study with this itch straight from hell was no easy task and some days I wanted to take a knife and cut and cut to rid myself of this horrific thing.

Eventually a new general practitioner arrived at my doctor's practice group. Young and very bright, he listened to all my pains and aches and voila, he said he thought he knew what was ailing me! He opened a thick journal and said, "Scleroderma," a name which in itself sounded scary. He referred me to a specialist for confirmation. Not knowing what scleroderma meant, I went to our on-site health practitioner and borrowed her medical dictionary. What I read confused me more!

The Internet gave me the opportunity to investigate and do some research. This was great in that I learned what was happening to me, but on the other hand it scared me stiff. Emotionally I was very low. I was in a new relationship with a widower who was still sensitive from his wife's death from a sudden illness two years earlier. This meant that I had to keep all this inside and try and work through my own shock and stress. When I eventually started being negative and a bit emotional, the support was not forthcoming, and I was still alone.

At least I knew that my new symptoms could be identified as the normal development of scleroderma. My face started showing signs of red blotches (telangiectasia) that ordinary makeup does not cover, so I had to go hunting for a foundation that could cover the spots, but at a premium cost, of course. At least makeup helps to keep the pretense going.

My mouth became much smaller. From time to time chewing became more difficult as my jaws developed painful spasms. Even a mouthful of water could start this! Swallowing became harder as drier foods tended to get stuck, so I would have to have a glass of water or liquid on hand to wash food down.

My hands became so tender in all the joints that a handshake became out of the question. Most people really like a firm handshake, which can reduce me to the feeling that at any moment I am apt to wet my pants. Bottles and tight jar lids are the most frustrating items! For the life of me I cannot open them. Coke bottles with the screw caps sometimes oblige, but mostly I have to find someone to assist me. This is one of the most irritating things for me, as I used to be the strong one who assisted others, and I could haul and carry heavy things with ease. Now I am helpless and constantly need to worry people for assistance.

My muscles are so useless that getting up from a squatting position is impossible without help or at least some support to grab and pull myself up. You should see me trying to get up from sitting on the floor! Like a toddler that just learned to walk, I first roll over on my knees, crawl to a support structure and then haul myself up, bit by bit. At least a sense of humor helps.

Raynaud's makes it difficult for me to work with anything clammy or cold, but washing has to be hung out and vegetables need to be prepared. Gloves help a lot and I have learned to use these as much as possible.

I used to garden a lot and loved the feeling of crumbling earth between my fingers. Now I dare not touch any weed or soil without the necessary protection for my hands or I suffer terrible itching and my hands crack open. That is also another painful experience, as these cracks are always on the fingers I use the most, and thus a continuous problem.

I have just applied for a new driver's license, for which fingerprints are taken. Eventually I had to get a doctor's letter to confirm that I have a skin problem and that the lines and cracks on my fingers are because of this. Now I have a driver's license card which states 'no prints'. (Does this mean I can perhaps have a new job? Shall we say, that of thief or any such one, seeing that I have no prints? Ha-ha!)

Lately reflux has become a constant problem for me, but thanks to my research, I sleep on my left side with good positive effect. I must say that reading some stories and researching scleroderma really has helped me to be able to manage my symptoms so much better!

In South Africa, scleroderma seems to be unknown as ninety-nine percent of people have not even heard of it. I hope that by establishing a web page with the help of the International Scleroderma Network, we can change this, thus enabling the people to come forward and share their stories, compassion, tips and give some emotional support to each other. We really need to get more awareness going around this disease. To try to explain to people what it is all about is really frustrating as they cannot understand or fathom all the aspects of scleroderma and what it does to you.

Five years after the itching started, I can see why most of the scleroderma patients say that the road until the proper diagnosis was made was the most difficult in some sense. We are made to feel like a fraud as different symptoms keep surfacing and we do not know what is going on.

Now that I do know, it is still hard to cope some days, as life seems to like throwing a curve ball. Other

SWAN SONG

When darkness closes
And rays of hope diminish
Turn around and look
To find the smallest speck
Of life's golden rays that's left
Take a good grip on it
Cherish every last bit
And it will brighten all
Your world that is left
Enhancing every flower and tree
And you and me.

days, when my energy levels are a bit better, the sun is shining brighter. I really appreciate things a lot more and I am trying hard to feel less stressed by daily problems. I do not always achieve success, but by constantly trying, I do make some progress.

Let us share our experiences and become a scleroderma family, knowing more about our bodies and how they work, than most other people. With lots of love and warm hugs to all the patients, caregivers, family and friends who make up our world.

◆ ❖ ◆

Rose Mainer
Texas, USA

I would like to thank the International Scleroderma Network for the valuable information, personal stories and the opportunity to connect with others with scleroderma. I have many friends and relatives here in the Houston area, but they can't understand this illness as well as my friends here.

I was finally correctly diagnosed with CREST after two years of thinking I was crazy. I did not have insurance until this year so I am finally on some medications that will hopefully help some. I am also involved with a research study at the local medical center and am trying to become more active in support groups. Time and energy are not my best attributes.

Right now the most pain I have is with finger ulcers and calcium deposits (calcinosis) on my elbows. Everything else has become a part of my life. I am learning to just take baby steps every day versus the fast-paced way I was living before.

I am interested in any home treatments or natural (herbal) alternatives for pain relief that anyone has had success with. I find myself taking too many pain pills because I am such a wimp when I am hurting; but of course that just worsens my stomach ulcer.

I am really looking forward to meeting new scleroderma friends. Take care.

◆ ❖ ◆

Rosemary Doolan
Australia

I was diagnosed in 1992 with a presence of positive anti-centromere antibodies (ACA). By 1997 I was unable to maintain paid work. To date there is no curative treatment.

Some of my symptoms may not be due to limited scleroderma; however most of these symptoms have appeared since my diagnosis. My Raynaud's began some twenty years ago and has been getting progressively worse; fingertip ulcerations occur regularly; and I have esophageal dysmotility with difficulty swallowing and gastric reflux. I had a laparoscopic Nissen Fundoplication in 2000. I also have sclerodactyly and thickening of facial skin with many telangiectasias on fingers, face, lips and tongue. I have alopecia areata. I have cardiac involvement as seen on my echocardiogram in 1998. I had a follow up echocardiogram in 2003, which showed no significant changes.

I suffer with pain and stiffness in muscles and joints due to thickening of tendons and joint linings. I have reduced lung function with impaired gas exchange, which was diagnosed by pulmonary function test (PFT) and CAT scan. The results are consistent with pulmonary vascular disease/lung parenchymal disease consisting of shortness of breath with activity, fatigue and generalized weakness.

I also have Sjögren's, which has caused dry mouth and dental problems, recurring mouth ulcers and dry nostrils. I have vitiligo on my hands, neck and face. I have occasional diarrhea/constipation due to thickening of the bowel wall, and mild anemia.

In November 1999, I developed mononeuropathy multiplex (bilateral perennial nerve palsies), which caused a mild right foot drop. In 1985, I presented with evidence of spondylitis from osteoarthritis. In 1991, right elbow tendonitis. In 1995, trochanteric bursitis in my left hip. In 1996, a trapezium was removed from my right thumb due to osteoarthritis. I have papules on my skin, mainly on upper back and forearms. They itch, and result in skin lesions from scratching.

I have been under the care of Dr. Laurie Clemens, who is a rheumatologist at St. Vincent's Hospital in Melbourne, since September 8, 2002. My general practitioner (GP) is Dr. R. Meyer in Mildura.

Update – January 2004

I started a scleroderma support group in Mildura, Victoria, Australia. If you or a loved one are affected by scleroderma or related illnesses or symptoms and live in our area, I invite you to contact me for meeting information.

Update – June 2004

My clinical features, including symptoms that may not necessarily be due to my scleroderma are as follows:
• Calcinosis of phalanges
• Raynaud's (began some twenty years ago) and has been getting progressively worse
• Fingertip ulceration occurring regularly
• Esophageal dysmotility; Atony of esophagus with gastric reflux and regurgitation
• Sclerodactyly; Skin thickening primarily of distal phalanges
• Flexion contracture right index finger
• Telangiectasias on fingers, hands, face, lips, tongue and inside nostrils
• Vitiligo on hands, neck and face
• Pulmonary arterial hypertension - shortness of breath with activity, fatigue
• Interstitial fibrosis of the lungs - impaired gas exchange (ventilation/perfusion mismatch)
• Dental problems (loose teeth) due to thickening of periodontal membrane and alteration of tooth suspensory ligament
• Dry mouth and nostrils
• Recurring mouth ulcers
• Diarrhea/constipation
• Alopecia areata
• Pruritus, primarily upper back, arms and hands
• Mononeuropathy multiplex (bi-lateral perennial nerve palsies), began in November 1999 with mild right foot drop
• Arthralgia - generalized, 1985
• Spondylitis identified, due to osteoarthritis, 1985
• Tendonitis, right elbow, 1991
• Left trochanteric bursitis, 1995
• Left olecranon bursitis, 2003

I am on many medications. The investigations that I have gone through are:

• Echocardiogram ~ 1998; 2003
• Nerve conduction studies ~ 1999 results consistent with mononeuropathy multiplex
• Esophageal manometry ~ 2000, results consistent with atony of the esophagus
• CAT scan/PFT scans ~ 1998; 2000; 2003 results consistent with pulmonary vascular disease/lung parenchymal disease

The treatments and surgery I have undergone are:

• In 2004 for an ulcer that progressed to osteomyelitis on second PIP joint, right index finger that was treated with intravenous medications.
• In 2003 for an infarction and dry gangrene of the right index finger.
• In 2000, gastroesophageal reflux disease alleviated with laparoscopic Nissen fundoplication surgery.
• In 1996 I had a trapezium resected from right thumb and in 1991, 1992, and 2003.
• In 2004 I had tendonitis in the right olecranon, which was treated with an injection, as well as bursitis in the left trochanter that was treated with injections and physiotherapy; and bursitis in the left olecranon.

◆ ❖ ◆

Sarah
Montana, USA

In 1991 my hands started swelling and my face was puffy in the morning. I did not go to a doctor then because it was intermittent.

By the summer of 1992 the swelling started to happen more often. My hands were sensitive to cold and getting contractures at the knuckles and were painful. My shoulders and hips were stiff and painful. I figured that it was arthritis and made an appointment with a rheumatologist. He did some tests. When the results came back he told me that it was CREST scleroderma. He prescribed a medication, but when I found out what the side effects were I told him that I did not want to take it. He did not explain what scleroderma was, so I went to the library and researched it. Boy, did that scare my husband and me! Needless to say, the doctor did not have a very good bedside manner!

I had up and down days but still did not want to take any medication. In March 1993 I learned that we now had a naturopathic doctor in town, and I went to see her. That was the best decision that I had made! She did a thorough exam and history. She put me on some herbs and vitamins. It took about three months, but the pain and swelling went away.

She had me see a rheumatologist, a cardiologist and a pulmonologist at different times to make sure everything was going alright. Everything went along fairly well until the fall of 2000, when my blood pressure went up. My naturopathic doctor tried herbs to control it but they just couldn't keep it down to an acceptable level. In March 2001 she had me go to the rheumatologist to see what he thought.

He prescribed an ACE inhibitor and I had a reaction to it. My hand swelled up, turned black and hurt so bad that it was an hour before I could even call his office. When I did call and told them what was going on, the nurse talked to the doctor and then advised me to cut the next dose in half and take an anti-inflammatory for the pain. Dumb me, I took another dose. I had to go to the emergency room. They took me right in and within ten minutes, had given me a shot for the pain. My blood pressure had skyrocketed.

They gave me something to counteract the ACE inhibitor. I was on morphine for eighteen months. I lost the tips of my baby finger and thumb. The other three fingers do not look very pretty, either. So my naturopathic doctor promised that I never had to go back to that rheumatologist. She sent me to my pulmonologist and he put me on another blood pressure medication.

I am maintaining now. I just went to a new rheumatologist and he is running some tests; creatine phosphokinase (CPK), bone scan, and echo-cardiogram. He was very concerned and kept looking at my hand and saying that it must have been very painful. I think he is a keeper!

I think it is very important to have a good working relationship with doctors. I feel that I am very fortunate with mine. My pulmonologist told me to call any time that I had a question and my naturopathic doctor gives me hugs!

Sari Hope Axelrod
Florida, USA

Nine years ago, at age forty, I was diagnosed with Raynaud's. This was in January, during a very cold Florida winter that was breaking records.

I was working at an engineering company sealing blueprints for building and zoning submittals, only to come home after work with blue fingers. At first I thought it was the dye in the ink from the blueprints on my fingertips, but I also noticed that my hair was falling out and I was losing weight as well. At this time I was also going through a divorce and working long, hard days as well as attending to my two children's needs. When I came home that night nine years ago to find my toes blue also, I knew my life would never be the same.

The next day after I showed my boss my fingers and toes, he sent me to my primary doctor who in turn sent me to a vascular specialist who confirmed in two days after blood tests that I had Raynaud's. I was put on steroids for a week as my fingers and toes were close to gangrene and amputation without circulation! After a week on steroids I was an emotional mess. I was then given the choice to spend the rest of my life on steroids or be treated as having angina, although my heart was well. I chose the blood thinners. My doctor and heart specialist still did not tell me about scleroderma.

During those first few years after being diagnosed with Raynaud's, I had to go to the grocery store with gloves on to reach into the frozen freezer. I would tell curious people who came up to me to inquire why I wore gloves in south Florida in the supermarkets that I was a burn victim and remind them not to play with matches.

As the years went on the symptoms progressed to CREST scleroderma and other effects of the illness. I have lost the ability to make saliva in my mouth and to make tears in my eyes. I am a patient of the Bascom Palmer Eye Institute in Miami, Florida, where they put punctal plugs into my tear ducts to make tears to cry. It was like having sprinklers inserted into my eyes for watering. But then they took them out and lasered my tear ducts closed in each eye to make the tears come. The worst part was smelling the flesh of my eyes being burnt as they were closed off.

I have lost nine teeth in the nine years because of the dry mouth problems and eat smaller meals because my esophagus is scarred because of reflux. The newest issue is that I tend to bleed from the slightest scratch for hours.

I recently attended dinner with family and friends and had ordered Florida stone crabs. The crabs were served cracked open, but somehow I caught my hand on the shell and started to bleed all over the table. I bled through the linen napkins and through several bandages as well. I have been taken off the blood thinners for awhile because my family is afraid that if I ever got into an accident that I might bleed to death. The doctors did not tell me about all these side effects, since each patient reacts to the illness differently.

Now I can laugh and be positive and proud to be able to talk openly about scleroderma. Living in Florida and with the constant air conditioning in all buildings, I have an amazing winter wardrobe. Everyone who knows me knows that I love gloves as a perfect gift and would love to have match-ing socks as well for my feet.

Now when people ask me if I am cold, with my winter clothes and gloves on in the summer of south Florida, I smile and tell them all about Raynaud's and scleroderma.

I am an advocate now, and last year I took on a diagnostic laboratory that was not calibrating antinuclear antibody (ANA) tests correctly. Through my persistence, I had them send my blood to Atlanta as they kept saying it was negative for ANA. I was actually getting worse and could not accept the negative results. I pursued it, and the laboratory had to notify the state of Florida of this revision and change their forms and calibrations.

Now I take blood thinners, saliva pills, antacids, and pain pills. I have worked all these years up until the last two months because of downsizing and the bad economy. No one else in my family has any of these health problems and since my middle name is Hope, I use my whole name, Sari Hope. I feel I was given this quirk or illness to raise the love and awareness of this autoimmune disease to the world. Bob Saget directed the movie *For Hope* about scleroderma, and I will spend the rest of my life fighting and talking to all the ignorant strangers who approach me daily, to make the world a 'warmer' place for those of us who are cold!

I am blessed with wonderful friends and family, and an amazingly positive attitude, but I have no significant other. The sad thing is that men get scared when they find out that I have this and they think I am going to die. I do not regret anything as I am blessed with so much more medical and spiritual awareness than most average people and I have a great appreciation for the love of life.

My specialist just asked me last week if I was going into politics, since I have a very strong determination to change American health care issues. I can only end this story with the fact that I have scleroderma, and it will never go away.

Good luck to all of us! Shalom!

CHAPTER 4

In Remembrance

Mom, your memory will never be forgotten.
I thank you for everything that you have done for me.
—Your ever loving son, Keith.

Introduction to Stories of Remembrance
by Tafazzul e-Haque Mahmud, M.D.

Dr. Mahmud is Assistant Professor and in charge of the Rheumatology Unit at Shaikh Zayed Federal Postgraduate Medical Institute, a teaching hospital in Lahore, Pakistan. He serves on the ISN Medical Advisory Board.

Like many of our scleroderma experts, the tragic death of a scleroderma patient inspired his dedication to rheumatology.

I was very good in cardiology during years of training in Pakistan and it was very much anticipated that I would specialize in it. I even completed my MD.

A new rheumatology clinic was being established at my hospital and they were looking for someone to run it on temporary basis until a new Registrar was appointed for the post. I was keen to take challenges, so I volunteered my name and that was the beginning of a new horizon in my medical life that changed everything altogether.

As I kept on working in that clinic, the level of misery that rheumatological patients suffer from became evident to me. I observed that all the world is spending resources to find better medical care for cardiac and stroke patients, but nothing significant was being done to find causes and treatments for rheumatological diseases; so much so that in a country like Pakistan, with over 120 million population, there was not a single physician dedicated to see and take care of such patients. All this continued to consolidate my urge to do something about it, and finally I decided to learn about rheumatology so that I could serve these suffering souls of my country.

I remember my first case of scleroderma, a young lady who when entered my clinic looked like one of Madam Tussaud's masterpieces. She entered my office gracefully, though I noticed her unease in walking and rapid breathing. She had "Wax-Mask Facies"; her facial skin was so tight that she was unable to speak properly.

She was twenty-two years of age and had been suffering from scleroderma for four years. She first noticed morning stiffness and fatigue, which her parents attributed to lot of hard work during her high school examination.

Gradually she noticed bluish discolouration of her fingers in the wintertime, which was often very painful. She described a strange feeling in her hands and over face while trying to wash them in the morning. She developed other features of the disease like hyperpigmentation, tightening of the skin, and digital infarcts.

Eventually she had to quit her education as she was always too tired to cope with stresses and she was unable to walk very far without becoming breathless. She also developed a feverish feeling that would stay all day long.

During the course of her illness she saw many physicians but her disease was not diagnosed. Initially it was attributed to depression, which she said she did develop—but that was only after listening to her physicians and other family members, because her complaints were being ignored by all of them. When the disease progressed further she was finally taken to a skin specialist who diagnosed her and referred her to me.

Well, there I was in my office with that miserable young lady who had already been told that there was no treatment for her disease and that there was nothing medicine can do to help her. She had advanced skin changes and frontal hair loss, signs of pulmonary hypertension, and Raynaud's.

On history she also revealed difficulty in swallowing food and occasional development of painful oral ulcers. I tried to reassure her that her condition would improve, but there was a strange question in her eyes that I could not answer.

I offered her admission to the hospital for management, which she reluctantly agreed to. During admission her investigations showed a very high erythrocyte sedimentation rate (ESR), strongly positive antinuclear antibodies (ANA), right heart strain pattern on echocardiogram (ECG), and a moderately high pulmonary artery pressure on Echo-doppler study.

That was all I could do as far her investigations were concerned. There was no facility for ENA profile estimation or for esophageal motility studies, and where such facilities were available they were too expensive for an ordinary person to afford.

Only skin biopsy for histological diagnosis was readily available, but her diagnosis was too obvious to require further confirmation. After discussing her cardiac status with the cardiologist, we began treatment for five days and her general condition started to improve. Subsequently, she was put on other medications as well.

She remained hospitalized for a week and I could see the ray of hope beginning to shine in her eyes. I was happy too, but at the same time I was worried about her pulmonary hypertension as there was no satisfactory treatment to offer. She gradually improved and most of her complaints subsided. Her Raynaud's and shortness of breath improved too, but not to my satisfaction.

She eventually got married but kept returning for follow up. I remember she was very happy when she disclosed her pregnancy. Her family was happy too. I could not predict at that point what might happen to her cardiac status with the pregnancy.

When she was near term, her husband contacted me because she was hospitalized at a private hospital with worsening shortness of breath. I went to see her, but it was too late. She was gasping for breath and I could sense the helplessness in her pleading eyes. Since she was rapidly deteriorating, her gynaecologist performed an emergency cesarean section to save the baby. As expected, she died on the operating table, but the baby girl was saved.

This tragic ending made me strong in my belief and determination to keep on working for patients with rheumatological diseases.

Here I am, so many years after her death, wondering whether the treatments that we have now for pulmonary hypertension would have saved her? And if diagnostic facilities were available then at a center without commercial motives, might we have saved her from progressing to pulmonary hypertension? Would she have lived to see her child and spend some more time with her family?

Of course, these are all "maybe's". We still have to go a long way to establish our unit further with modern facilities to diagnose and treat such patients. With limited resources and means, I don't know how long will it take—but I am determined to keep trying!

Anghelita
Aunt Lia's Scleroderma
Italy

This story was translated from Italian to English by Kevin Howell. He is a Clinical Scientist for Professor Carol Black at the Royal Free Hospital in London. The Italian version of this story is in Chapter 10.

I am the niece of Aunt Lia, who unfortunately is no longer here with us. Her disease was very distressing and rapidly-progressing, and from the date of her diagnosis she lived only three months. They were months of suffering for her and for all of us, and above all for her daughters, aged sixteen and eighteen.

I want to remember her for her cheerfulness and joy of living. She was forty-six years old and she was pretty, with a smile that touched the heart.

Her disease began with ulcers on the fingers. Then there was a thickening and pallor of the face, and little by little the whole body. Then it entered inside and struck her kidneys, and she started to have dialysis. Then it affected her heart, and in the end her death was caused by lung failure.

I will never forget her face. She was suffering but she was affectionate with everyone. This happened in 1984 when I was a little girl. The memory of Aunt Lia is always with me.

Keith
In Memory of My Mom
Delaware, USA

In fall of 1982 my mom was diagnosed with this dreadful disease and it caused kidney failure. My mom had a kidney transplant in February 1988.

I was stationed in Korea, but was able to be home in Miami the day after the transplant. Then in the summer of 1994, her kidneys failed again.

After that incident my mom was able to carry on a productive life but her illness continued to get worse. In January 1996 I decided to move from Baltimore, Maryland, back to Miami, Florida, so that I could look after her in her time of need, giving up everything for her.

I have enjoyed the last three years we were able to spend with each other. She was a single mother raising one child, whom she raised very well. After entering the hospital on February 15, 1999, she was diagnosed with lung problems, but due to the scleroderma her blood pressure could not be maintained by her own body. My mom passed away of respiratory failure on February 25, 1999, four days after my 33rd birthday.

Luckily I was able to share this time with her and I thank God for that. The thing that hurts the most is that she will never be able to meet her first grandchild, who is due on May 26, 1999.

So tell that special person how much you love them if you have not done so, because tomorrow is not promised. I was lucky to tell her how much I loved her. My mother was the best friend and the best parent that anyone could ever have.

Mom, your memory will never be forgotten. I thank you for everything that you have done for me. Your ever loving son, Keith.

◆❖◆

Linda Weller
In Memory of My Mother, Barbara "Bobbi" Bast, 1947-2003
Wisconsin, USA

All she wanted was for others to learn of this disease and know her story. She requested this about two weeks before she died on October 24, 2003.

Barbara or "Bobbi" as she liked to be called, was diagnosed with CREST in 1990. She had major joint pain on a regular basis along with other symptoms, bowel problems and a lot of pain. After doing some reading about CREST syndrome she (and eventually her doctor) realized she had scleroderma. The worst of it seemed to have started with having a knee replacement, then a new kneecap, as they had put the wrong size in the first time. Healing was very slow for her. As time went on she developed a sore on her elbow that did not heal, so they removed part of her elbow. Her fingers started getting sores that would not heal, so five of her fingers were amputated, at different times.

Then she had a second knee replacement, the other one this time. Another sore started and would not heal, so again the doctors decided to remove the parts that did not heal. She was on so many medications! She was placed in a nursing home after that knee surgery. She started to get involuntary shakes in her arms and legs and was embarrassed by this. Her kidneys and liver were starting to fail also. She developed a bad infection on the knee, so they decided to remove the artificial knee and put spacers in so that maybe the infection would go away.

Mom then had a colonoscopy and when she came out of recovery the next day her small intestine started to bleed and they could not stop it. She was put in intensive care, and given five units of blood. The doctors told my family that we should decide if she would want to keep fighting or not.

After so many years of constant pain, she had been saying all along that she did not want to live like this. So we stopped everything; the pills, the blood, everything, and let her body decide when to go. She was kept comfortable on pain medication until the end. The infection finally got to her lungs. She died with her husband, her two daughters and her son at her side. My mom was the strongest person I have ever known.

Mom, I hope this helps and in some small way is what you wanted me to do for you. There are so many details only you could really explain. I love you and miss you so much.

Lori
A Tribute to My Dad, Leo
Massachusetts, USA

Do you ever wonder what makes a good dad? Well, let me tell you about mine. Since the time I was a very little girl, I thought my dad was the greatest. He would play with me whenever I asked, whether it be a board game, baseball, fishing or anything. One of the things I remember most was when he would fly me around like an airplane. He would lay on his back with his feet in the air, and my little body on top of his legs and he would 'fly' me and my brother around. I remember it being so much fun!

As we got older, my brother and I were involved in many sports and each time we looked up into the stands, there he was, even when it was an away game. We were not the best athletes, but we tried hard and he never criticized us whatsoever. He just gave us the encouragement we needed. He continued to follow this pattern with his four grandchildren: Ryan, Jeff, Allison and Nicole. They loved him so very much and he just adored them all, for they were his pride and joy! He was such a devoted, active participant in their lives as a 'Papa', just as he was a father to me and my brother, Jim, and a husband to my mother, Carol.

My dad also was a very hard worker. He worked at Texas Instruments for thirty-nine years, and retired almost two years ago. Little did he know he would never get to enjoy it. He did not even live five months past his sixtieth birthday.

Now let me tell you about his history with the horrible disease, scleroderma. He began to notice symptoms in 1989, the year my brother and I both got married. He was working in the yard one day, pulling up weeds and when he came in the house, he complained of his hands being puffy. He thought it was from pulling the weeds and such. When the puffiness did not go away, he went to his doctor. His doctor said he might have Raynaud's phenomenon, but never gave him any information regarding scleroderma and how this could be related.

He continued on, not worrying too much about his hands, and we made it through the weddings in June and then again in October. We had made plans to go to Atlantic City that April, but we never got there. My father had hypertension for many years, but he had been doing so well that his doctor had taken him off of his medications.

One day while at work, he did not feel right and went to the nurse. She took his blood pressure and it was sky-high. She sent him immediately to his doctor, who actually asked if it could be due to stress! That night, he got into bed early and still felt horrible. We called his doctor and they said to get him to the hospital as soon as possible. Come to find out, the blood pressure was due to a renal crisis from the scleroderma. We found this out after a few days in the hospital, and many tests. When the doctor told us it was scleroderma, we had no idea what he was talking about. They said it was a rare disorder, and that there was no cure, but we had no idea how bad it could be. My mom and I did research and were horrified to learn what a devastating disease this could be. Our family was in shock.

After this renal crisis, my dad's looks changed. He had been very robust and healthy-looking, with so much energy and zest for life. He changed by looking a bit more wasted, his neck skin tightened a bit as did his face, but not so much that people thought he was ill; they just thought he had lost some weight. He did not have as much energy any more, but over time, his kidney function had stabilized and he had regular check-ups and was told he was doing fantastic. The doctors told him the renal crisis was probably the worst that would happen to him. He did remain stable and did great for about ten years, though his hands were a bit worse, more hardened and such, making it more difficult for him to do some things.

Time had gone on and he now had four beautiful grandchildren. Ryan was born in 1992 and was the apple of my dad's eye, and Ryan just adored him. They had so much fun together, they would just play games, go places together, and they had developed a great bond. Ryan really looked forward to seeing him, and we saw him almost every day since we lived so close by. Then my brother and his wife had Jeff two years after and then came along Allison and then, Nicole. All the kids loved playing with Papa. He taught them all to swim in their in-ground pool.

As I look back now on all the times we spent together, whether it just was hanging out or vacationing or at holidays, it makes me very happy and proud to have such a close-knit family. We truly enjoyed being together and had a lot of fun, and I find this comforting.

In May 2001, we had a big retirement party for my dad. He had worked so hard, he deserved a nice party with his family and friends. But after having had a routine CAT scan to see how his lungs were doing, the doctors discovered a huge kidney tumor and things took a turn for the worse. This was in June 2001.

In August 2001, after an agonizing two months of waiting, the surgeons finally removed what turned out to be renal cell carcinoma. The good news was it was totally contained and my father would not need to undergo chemotherapy or radiation. We hoped his other kidney would be able to handle the workload, and were so happy that he seemed he would be able to recover and get on with his retirement!

He recovered pretty nicely with no major complications, but he seemed to be getting very short of breath on exertion, especially with climbing stairs. He thought it was his heart as he also had a stent placed due to a blockage a few years prior. So he reluctantly went back to his doctor again. They ruled out any type of blockage or heart problem, and after undergoing some more testing (an echocardiogram and an MRI), they sent him to a pulmonologist as they believed this time it was his lungs that were getting progressively worse. It was true, they were worse. He had moderate pulmonary hypertension along with pulmonary fibrosis and inflammation in his lungs from the scleroderma.

I have read many articles that state people with scleroderma have progression after undergoing surgery and I truly believe this is what happened to my father, since after he had his kidney out he seemed to go progressively downhill.

There was really no treatment for this, except for some therapies that were believed might help. This included a daily dose of corticosteroids, blood thinners, and cyclophosphamide (Cytoxan). Cyclophosphamide is a very powerful drug that suppresses the immune system; it is an oral chemotherapy treatment. When you are on this medication, you are supposed to be on a prophylactic antibiotic also so you will not get a dreaded pneumonia called pneumocystis carinii pneumonia (PCP). This is seen in many AIDS patients when their immune system is very compromised and sometimes in cancer patients who are on chemotherapy.

Unfortunately, my parents were not told of the great risks of this medication. They were told his biggest worry would be possible blood in his urine and maybe bladder cancer on down the road. He was never told about PCP. Also, he was intolerant to the sulfa antibiotics, so his doctor decided to hold the antibiotics for the time being, again never telling him of the risk of this pneumonitis! He never would have decided to take this medication if he truly knew all of the risks involved.

My father also had a great deal of difficulty on the blood thinner. They just could not get the right dosage for him. His blood was either way too thin, or not thin enough to be doing him any good. This was a major source of anxiety and frustration for everyone, but especially for my father, as he was at the hospital every other day having his blood drawn.

By the summer of 2002, although he had many problems, he was trying to adjust and enjoy the summer. However, because of his physical limitations due to the shortness of breath and the aggravation with the many blood draws, he was becoming very discouraged. I believe he knew he was getting worse, but really never complained about how bad he really was feeling. Although we were worried, we thought it was just progression of his disease, not pneumonia.

It was the beginning of August, 2002, when suddenly my maternal grandmother dropped dead at age ninety-one. My parents were busy caring for my elderly grandfather and although my father never complained, he himself was close to death.

The night of my grandmother's funeral, dad had the chills so bad that he could not get warm. He was sweating and becoming more short of breath, but did not complain so much that he needed to go to the hospital. The next morning I stopped in to see him and he looked terrible and was shaking and was very short of breath. I called his doctor immediately as my mother was at church with my grandfather. His doctor said to bring him into the hospital. He warned me on the phone that since my father was on chemotherapy, he was at risk for very rare infections. This was the first I had heard of this.

We got him to the hospital and they placed him on fifty percent supplemental oxygen and did a lot of tests. When his doctor saw him, he said he would put him on antibiotics, hoping it was bronchitis, and actually released him from the hospital. PCP cannot be diagnosed without a bronchoscopy.

He went home, but he did not feel any better, and in fact, he felt much worse. He had severe shortness of breath and my mother drove him to the hospital in the wee hours of the morning, only one and a half days after being sent home on the antibiotic. At the hospital, he was immediately placed on oxygen and they again ran a battery of tests and blood work. They also had to do the bronchoscopy to rule out the PCP. After the bronchoscopy, he needed to be placed on more oxygen and his oxygen saturation levels were still dropping. We were encouraged by the doctors as they had him on every antibiotic imaginable to cover any type of infection he might have and were told it might be several days before he would begin to improve. The doctors at this point suspected PCP, but the bronchoscopy report never grew out anything, probably because they had placed him on some antibiotics in the meantime. But he was septic, having the disease throughout his body now, and he never did improve. That night he was placed on oxygen, but his saturation levels dropped even further and he could not catch his breath.

He had to be rushed to the intensive care unit (ICU) and intubated, which must have been even more horrific for him than it was for us having to watch this and not being able to help him. This was the last time we saw him awake, since after they did this procedure he had to be very heavily sedated to not fight the respirator.

He was in ICU for many days and got progressively worse, needing dialysis and so many other things I cannot even remember, as I was in such shock seeing him like that. He did not look like the same person. He was bloated and had tubes sticking out of him everywhere. To this day, I still cannot believe that was my father lying in that hospital bed. My only comfort is hoping that he felt no pain since he was heavily sedated.

We are sure there were many things he would have liked to have said to his family before he died. He was such a family man and truly enjoyed all the little things in life such as taking a walk, taking pride in his house and yard, and cherishing his family.

Since there was no hope for my father, as his lungs were severely infected, we had to take him off the respirator. They took out all the tubes and we gathered around him at his bedside. We held his hands and told him how much we loved him and watched him take his last breath at 5:50 p.m. on September 6, 2002.

It has been a rough year for our family, but I wanted to write this to possibly help anyone else out there who may be going through this. Take every precaution, educate yourself and above all, look out for yourself as the doctors may tell you one thing, but do what is right for you. You, above all, know how you are feeling and if it is not right, you must insist on further treatment.

◆ ❖ ◆

Michele Crowder
In Loving Memory of My Father
New York, USA

I have a story to tell that is very sad to me. I lost my father this summer on July 28, 2004, to a very rare and horrible disease. I have been having the worst time dealing with his loss and thought that it might help me, and possibly someone else, to tell his story.

My dad was diagnosed only four months prior to his death with CREST Syndrome.

He often suffered with puffy hands, pain, and joint stiffness. Just this past winter he had some breathing problems and had tests done. While he was going through all these tests and seeing specialists, they came to the conclusion that he had this rare but livable disease called CREST Syndrome. He was doing well and it was manageable. I got the impression that he did not think this disease was a big issue. He would often joke, laugh and make fun of his disease.

Then about a month after his diagnosis he ended up in the hospital with a bad case of pneumonia. It was now evident that the scleroderma from the CREST had started to affect his lung function. As before, my dad was able to handle all of this with a joke or two. I guess that is how he comforted himself through his very short but difficult journey with this disease.

Upon departing from his first hospital visit with this disease, he was ordered to use oxygen all the time, and to return for chemotherapy treatment. He was also given a prescription for steroids. Although he did not want to be seen with the oxygen, he did the best he could to use it. He did not use it all the time, but enough to sustain his oxygen at a normal level. Also, he seemed to do well with his chemotherapy and medications. He lost a lot of weight and appeared to be weak at times, but he was able to hold down his coaching job that he loved so much.

About two months after that hospital stay he had chemotherapy again. This time the treatments made him sick and the steroids kept him up nights with agitation. He seemed to suffer for about two weeks before he felt better.

Then he had testing done for lung function. He left me a voicemail message about the results from the tests. On the message he was so happy that he cried because all was going well with him. I guess he was scared that he may have gotten worse and he did not want me to know it. He seemed overjoyed and confident that this disease did not get the best of him, which made me very happy.

About a week later he came down with shingles. The doctor treated the virus with antibiotics and stopped his steroids. We all felt that shingles was not a big deal. We figured it was nothing compared to what had been happening to him the past few months. My dad looked terrible and I knew in my gut that something was wrong. I did extensive research on the Internet as I have been doing regarding CREST, and I did not find anything that seemed bad about having shingles, so I did not worry about it.

A few days later, my parents drove upstate about seven hundred miles (to my father's hometown of Brockport, New York) for a family reunion. On the day of the reunion my dad talked to family and friends about death. Surprising to no one, he spoke about his last wishes and thoughts; but surprising to everyone was that that night he went to the hospital with breathing problems. It seemed as if the scleroderma in his lungs was creating a problem again.

After two days in the hospital undergoing tests, there seemed to be nothing wrong except his lung function, which was excellent just two week prior, and possible problems with the shingles. On that day, I was notified that he was in the hospital and I had the chance to speak to him. He reassured me that everything was okay and he was doing well. He wanted to know how we were doing, since we were seven hundred miles away from him, and he spoke with my three small children. I was hoping that would lift his spirits and I think it did. We ended our phone conversation with "I love yous".

The next morning I got the call that he had gone into septic shock and was not doing well. I gathered our things and we all got in the car and drove up there as fast as we could. Upon our arrival I was unsure of what was taking place. I did not know that what I was about to be dealing with would be so difficult. I was hoping to get there and we all could cheer him up, especially his grandchildren, but that was not the case. As I walked in the quiet and dim lighted hospital room I was in shock to see my dad lying there lifeless! He was in an induced coma due to difficult breathing from a massive heart attack that occurred that morning.

My brother and I stayed the night with him so our mother could get some rest. I watched, touched and felt nothing but lifeless sadness as he lay there in that bed. I knew it was bad when he started to burn with fever during the night and I knew I would have to accept whatever had to be.

The next morning we had to make some very difficult decisions regarding resuscitation and also letting him go. It seemed as if his systems had started to shut down quickly, so my brother and I decided to let him go quietly and peacefully. I had problems with that and I still do now, but inside I know it was for the best. He suffered so much horror and then happiness, and I think he knew he was dying inside. For my own selfish reasons I wanted to keep him alive and in my heart I knew that was wrong, so I had to let my daddy go.

I am going through a very rough time right now dealing with his death and that is why I am writing this story. I want to try to help myself and if I can help someone else in the process, then I know my dad has touched another life! He was so loved. I never knew how many others loved and appreciated my dad as much as I did.

My wish is that all of you have success in fighting this horrifying disease. I do not know why things happen to us in this world, but I am working on believing that things happen for a reason. My prayer is that my experience with my father's death will help someone else.

Raymond Girouard
In Memory of My Mother, Claudia Girouard
Canada

It was the most beautiful death that you could ever imagine.

On September 31, 2002, my mother, Claudia Girouard, lost her courageous fight with scleroderma.

In 1994, my mother felt pain in her arms and the doctors could not figure out what it was. She went for test after test and the only thing the doctors could say was arthritis.

One day she fainted. The skin on her arms turned brown. Needless to say, that really confused the doctors. Back she went for more tests, until finally they got it right and diagnosed her with scleroderma.

When the doctor diagnosed my mother with scleroderma my family could only ask, "What is that?" We did not have a clue what it was, and to be honest, the doctors could not tell us either. No one could tell us anything.

We did not know what was in store for my mother. We did not know how rough it was going to be or how dangerous scleroderma really is. Thanks to many wonderful web sites on scleroderma we eventually found the answers we were looking for.

From the time she first fainted and her arms turned brown, we started to see significant changes in her appearance. My mother was a big beautiful lady when first diagnosed, and became a very small and very pitiful looking lady when she passed on.

During her illness she never complained once. She never complained that she could not swallow or even that her lungs were only working at forty percent. All she wanted to do was live.

I was a single dad to a very wonderful son and my mother helped me every chance she could. She cooked until her fingers started to curl and she could no longer hold a spoon. She loved to laugh and loved being involved in our lives and with her grandchildren. My mother did not stop living during her illness. She went to every family gathering and any benefit to support others.

Many times during her illness there were battles. She had three heart attacks. Every cold she got was a battle. Her blood pressure would go down and have a hard time getting back up. But she would bounce right back up and get on to another journey.

The final three years of my mother's life, I must say, were the worst three years of my life. I had a very hard time accepting the changes in my mom's appearance and her life. I would not go to my parents' house to see her, because every time I looked at her I mourned.

One day, with just her and I at home, I sat with my mother and told her why I had such a hard time visiting and we made peace. I told her how I felt and how much it hurt me to see her this way. She just looked at me and called me a coward and laughed. But she understood and thanked me.

In September 2002, my mother started to notice her toes were turning black. My sister brought my mother to the hospital. She was admitted right away. Over the next two months she lost both big toes. After each surgery she got weaker and weaker. Then the doctors noticed that one of her toes was not healing and it looked like another operation was in store for her. But first they had to fix her feeding tube that moved during her time there.

Every day in the hospital my mom was getting weaker. Before the doctors operated on the second toe my mother cried, fearing that she was not going to wake up from the operation. Well, she did wake up. She woke up to more suffering and more pain than what she had before.

During the days before the final operation on my mother's feeding tube, the doctor went to her and asked her if she wanted it done. He did not hold back and was honest and told her that there was a very strong chance she was not going to make it. She was weak and her blood pressure was very low. She looked at the doctor and told him that she could not go on like this anymore and was ready for her place beside God, who she believed in very much.

The night before the operation she asked the family to pray to God that he would take her. That night that is what we all did. We all went to bed that night and we wished for what my mother asked. On that night I was working out of town and I did not want to be anywhere near that hospital. I stayed in my motel room and just prayed. I hoped that when I got into work that morning that I would have a message to call home and it would finally be over. But that just was not meant to be. Her operation was postponed for a couple of hours. Every one of her brothers and sisters, all sixteen of them, and six of her children, except me, the big coward, was there.

Before the operation my mother asked everyone in and said good-bye to each of them. She apologized to my dad for being sick and told him to take care of us all. She told everyone that she loved them and told everyone to take care.

When they came to get her for her operation she looked at her mother and her sister right in the eye and she asked them to pray that she does not come back. During the operation the chapel in the hospital was full of people praying for this wonderful lady who had so much strength and courage. They prayed that the Lord would finally make peace with her and take her home.

She made it through the operation. They brought her upstairs to her room where she could be with her family. An hour later my mother was finally called to her place in heaven. It was the most beautiful death that you could ever imagine. She got to say good-bye before the end.

After her death I made it a personal goal to make people aware of scleroderma in Canada. I have been emailing the government and have also been in contact with the scleroderma groups in Canada. I have been asking the government to support funding for research, and to educate the doctors and families of patients who are suffering from this horrid disease. I also made a web page entitled, "In Memory of My Mom."

Now my mother's brother, my Uncle Edmond, has just been diagnosed with scleroderma, and a new battle begins.

Update – March 2003

Uncle Edmond is doing fine and he is still going strong. Just like his father, in my eyes, he walks on water. He is a wonderful man and a very caring father.

But now another case has showed up in our family. My Uncle John, who is also a very wonderful man, was told this week that he also has scleroderma.

Coincidence? I think not. The doctors here tend to think so. My mother was fifty-two when she was told she had scleroderma and her brothers are also in their fifties.

It is very scary to think what may be happening here. When my mother got scleroderma, my family had no clue what to expect. We did not know the changes that were going to take place with her, but for my uncle that is not the case as they have seen it.

Now we have to put our heads together and try to work on what we have to do to keep them with us. My mother has ten other brothers and sisters. I know how scared I am for my three wonderful children, Nathan, Derek and Kim. Could you imagine how they feel? I know they are scared, too.

I feel like I am just waiting to hear the doctor tell me I have it.

I have three wonderful aunts who were with my mom the whole time, and I know they will be there for my uncles also. For now all we can do is pray. Pray that they find a cure for this horrid illness. And I pray for every one who is suffering with it. May God give you all strength and the courage to fight this and beat it. Do not let this get the best of you.

I plan on being a voice against scleroderma. I will speak to those who matter and who I believe can help make a difference.

Rodger Mansfield
Missouri, USA

Many of you may know the moment. That first time that your loved one says, "I had a strange cough. I feel a bit different today." I can vividly recall the moment when my wife Kathleen said those words to me just four years ago. It was the first cough that was not "right". The first time that she knew something was wrong. Little did we know how wrong.

We learned that there would many firsts: the first doctors visit; the first biopsy; the first difficult treatment choice; the first time we knew what we faced. The first of what would be many firsts.

Fortunately, Kathleen was able to get a quick and accurate diagnosis of diffuse scleroderma. Unfortunately, despite the best medical care, despite our best personal efforts to learn about this condition and to make all of the right choices, Kathy lost her battle this summer. It was fours years to the day that she had that first cough.

Kathy never asked why this terrible disease happened to her, nor was she ever bitter about it. Rather, she asked what she could learn. She learned how to make the most of every day. She and I also learned that we live in a mortal, frail and imperfect world which is not fair. Knowing that helped us to move forward during the past four years. We loved each other and made the most of everything we did together. We had few regrets.

But I have also learned many things over the past four years from Kathleen, such as how to be kinder, gentler, a better father and husband, more faithful and a better human being. And most importantly, how to live each day as if it is your last and to think carefully about your words and deeds.

As we think about how this happened, I encourage you to talk about life and death issues with your spouse, your family and your doctors. If you have specific wishes, you need to have them legally documented, and made known to those who can help you and ensure that those around you can be strong enough to see it through. Trust me, this is not easy.

So how do we move on with a whole lot of more firsts in our lives? We have also moved on by establishing the *Kathleen M. Mansfield Foundation: Building a Better Community Through Knowledge, Leadership and Service.* This is a foundation to promote Kathleen's love of community service. It gives us great comfort to continue her work. We also created a web site, *The Kathy Report,* that allows us to share more information about scleroderma and its many complications.

◆❖◆

Samantha L. Lindgren
In Memory of My Mother
North Dakota, USA

My mother died on March 18, 1996, from complications of scleroderma. For several years before her actual diagnosis of scleroderma, she was suspected of having an enlarged heart. Next, was the numbness in her extremities, which was occurring at the same time. She was told to carry on and that they would find out the cause. She was placed on heart medication and blood pressure medication. I do not think they really had an explanation for the numbness.

My mother had worked hard all her life with jobs that ranged from bartending at nights to housekeeping during the days at a local motel. When 1994 rolled around she was developing ulcers at the tips of her fingers, which happened in the winter. She thought that maybe she had frostbite. The ulcers would disappear, but only momentarily. They began to return more frequently. She began to notice her hands were not only cold all the time, but were sensitive to touch and cold.

My mother worked with her hands so for her to cut back on work hours was a real sacrifice for her. In 1995, she noticed her symptoms were beginning to include weight loss, fatigue, blood pressure changes, retention of water, and an overall change in who she was.

On December 23, 1995, she was advised to check into the hospital, but her favorite holiday, Christmas, was just around the corner and she was not going to miss that for the world. On December 26, 1995, she was admitted to the hospital in Minot, North Dakota. She had so many tests that they were beginning to wear her down. She had one last test that would leave her recovering in the intensive care unit (ICU). When she awoke they had her diagnosis of scleroderma, which none of us had ever heard of before. We would soon find out the wrath it had planned for her. The doctor explained everything well for us, but the word that dumbfounded us was fatal.

She was only forty-five years old. How did this happen? Why her? Nobody could and has never been able to say anything else except that, "It was God's plan."

The last few months of my mother's life I was not really around her except during her next hospitalization, where I spent day and night with her like I did in Minot. This time we were in Bismarck. They ran more tests on her and before one procedure she told me to put on my headphones and give her my hand. I had my headphones turned as high as they would go and I felt her squeeze my hand and heard a scream like no other. Her blood vessels were beginning to collapse because of the blood thinner she was on, and they could not switch the IV to the other arm because of this. She was poked over twelve times with the needle and once I remember seeing the nurse move the needle around in her arm to find a vein.

It is the time I spent alone with her that I remember most. I thought that I had already lost my mother due to her limitations, but I found she was still there, a crazy, middle-aged woman and an unbelievable night owl. I found out how much like her I really was. After she was discharged from the hospital it was my aunts who were there for her and supporting her, while I was out literally raising hell. I always dwell on that because had I known that a month after her discharge she would be gone, I would have been with her all the time.

The night before she died I remember she was sleeping on the couch while I was watching television in the living room. Out of a sound sleep she sat straight up and said, "What in the hell are you watching?" I told her it was an Aaron Spelling soap and after that she went back to sleep. I was up late that night and when I walked by the living room I contemplated whether to either go lie by her or stay up with her. I did neither for the fear of her reminding me that I was up too late for a school night and I would catch hell if she knew. So I crept by her and looked in one more time and whispered, "Good night. I love you mom."

I woke up to my mom's sister knocking on my door frantically saying that there was something wrong with my mom. I ran into the living room and my mom was rolling around on the couch while my grandmother tried to console her. My aunt tried to get hold of a physician in town and he told us to wait for the Indian Health Service to open up. I suggested that we call another doctor whom he practiced with. The doctor said she would be ready and that we had to come by her house, which was two and a half blocks away, and she would follow us in her vehicle back to our house.

I remember walking back into our house and my grandma told us to be quiet because my mother was finally resting. They told me to take a quick shower and to pack a bag because I was going to ride with her in the ambulance. I took no longer than four minutes to dress. When I returned to the living room I walked in just in time to hear, "I am sorry. There is nothing more we can do."

My mom began her new journey at 7 a.m. that Monday morning. I know she is still with me because since then only good things happen on Mondays. My oldest child was born on a Monday at 7:15 p.m., and my youngest was born on a Monday at 7:21 p.m.

Susan Raby-Dunne
In Memory of My Mother
Canada

My mother was diagnosed with scleroderma around 1970. She was taken around to meet a couple of scleroderma patients and told this was what she could expect. They were bedridden and unable to feed or care for themselves. She refused that prediction and vowed she would not allow the disease to disable her.

She began to meditate faithfully using the transcendental meditation (TM) program twice a day without fail. She also changed her diet to mostly whole grain and vegetarian foods. She began to drink several glasses of water daily.

The effects she suffered from scleroderma were hardening of her fingers and toes and extreme sensitivity to cold and touch. If she got the slightest bit chilled, her fingers and toes would turn white and she would have to run hot water on them to restore circulation. If she stubbed her toes or banged her fingers on anything the pain was excruciating. Her facial skin became very drawn. She could not totally close her mouth to where you could not see her teeth. She also had digestive problems.

In spite of those symptoms, she lived a fairly full and productive life for over thirty years after her diagnosis. She danced with my father and they were accomplished ballroom dancers. She painted and played golf until she was eighty years old.

About two years ago, she began to fail. She had serious digestive troubles, heart irregularities and a minor stroke. She died October 15th, 2002, at the age of eighty-four. She weighed less than seventy pounds.

If she had taken her doctor's prediction for her imminent demise to heart in 1970, she would have packed it in long ago. From what I have read, I am not sure which type of scleroderma she had. It seems to be a combination of several types. She was a fighter and was able to live well with the disease. I think her attitude and belief were the most important factors in her survival.

◆ ❖ ◆

PART 2

Juvenile and Localized Scleroderma

CHAPTER 5

Juvenile Scleroderma

She has gone through a lot,
but she has never asked,
"Why me?".

—Debra Reynolds

Juvenile Scleroderma
by Fernanda Falcini, M.D.

Dr. Fernanda Falcini is a Pediatric Rheumatologist in the Department of Pediatrics, University of Florence, Italy.

Main Types of Juvenile Scleroderma: Localized and Systemic

Q: My child has been diagnosed with scleroderma. Is this the same as scleroderma that occurs in adults? Is the disease outcome as dreadful as in adults or is juvenile scleroderma a different illness?

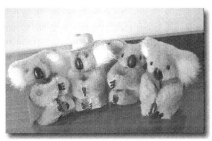

(L-R) Two Main Types of Scleroderma
1. Localized (Morphea, Linear)
2. Systemic (Limited, Diffuse)

The very first thing you need to know is what type of scleroderma is affecting your child, since the term "juvenile scleroderma" is applied to both localized scleroderma and systemic sclerosis (SSc).

There is a big difference between the localized or systemic forms of scleroderma concerning disease course, therapy, long-term complications, and outcome. Localized scleroderma—such as morphea or linear—is by far the most common type of scleroderma in children. Systemic scleroderma (SSc) is extremely rare in childhood.

Localized Scleroderma: Morphea and Linear

Juvenile localized scleroderma is a distinct entity that may be differentiated from juvenile systemic sclerosis by being confined to skin with rare, though possible, internal organ involvement.[1]

Localized scleroderma is most common in children, whereas systemic is most common in adult-onset scleroderma.

Among all admissions to pediatric rheumatology units for connective tissue diseases, localized scleroderma accounts for 2% of the patients. Although it remains a rare condition, skin hardening changes in your child could signify morphea or linear scleroderma.

The cause (etiology) and development (pathogenesis) of localized scleroderma are still unknown. Infections and trauma often seem to be associated with the appearance of skin alterations in children, but autoimmunity certainly plays a role, as confirmed by the presence of antinuclear antibodies in some patients.

Only very rarely (from 0% to 2% of cases), do localized symptoms develop into systemic scleroderma.[1] So once your child has been diagnosed with localized scleroderma by a physician experienced in scleroderma, there is a 98% to nearly 100% chance that it will not ever progress to the systemic form.

Recent research from a large multinational study indicates that about 25% of children with localized scleroderma will develop one or more symptoms besides just skin involvement. However, the additional symptom(s) or antibodies do not mean that the child will progress to full-fledged systemic sclerosis.[5] The subset of children with morphea or linear who are at risk for eventually progressing to systemic are those who also have prominent Raynaud's and anti-centromere antibodies (ACA); even then, it is just a posssibility and not a certainty.[3]

Thus, about 75% of children with localized will not develop even one symptom outside of their morphea or linear skin involvement, and 98% or more will not have any risk of developing systemic scleroderma. However, even this very slight risk may still seem uncomfortably high for those who are understandably worried about systemic scleroderma.

To put things into perspective, at least 1 out of 3 children will develop cancer in their lifetime, and many more will eventually succumb to heart disease. Since we are all accustomed to living with such risks, most patients and family members can take things in stride, once the imagined versus the real and relative risks posed by scleroderma are plainly acknowledged and explained.

Different subtypes of localized scleroderma are recognized, and each requires a different therapeutic approach. The main subtypes are:

A. Morphea (Plaque and Generalized)

B. Linear (including En Coupe de Sabre, and Parry-Rombergs)

A. Localized Scleroderma: Morphea

Plaque morphea is the most common form of localized scleroderma. It begins with an oval area of hard skin (induration) that is ivory-colored and surrounded by a violet or purplish (violaceous) border (halo).

Morphea plaques typically occur on the trunk. The arms, legs, and face are usually spared. Over time, the plaques may become atrophied, and either lighter or darker than they were at first; sometimes turning pink, brown, or gray. Morphea is defined as generalized in a patient who has many areas of morphea, or when several plaques join together to cover a large area.

Morphea may regress spontaneously in most children over a period ranging from 2 to 5 years. Children with plaque morphea that is not spreading or affecting the underlying muscle or bone usually don't need anything more than local creams as emollients. They should avoid local stress and sun exposure. Residual hyperpigmentation may be the only cosmetic concern.

B. Localized Scleroderma: Linear

Linear scleroderma usually begins during childhood or adolescence, typically in children under 8 years old. The estimated prevalence is 50 per 100,000 in children under 17 years of age.

It starts with an area of tight skin on an arm or leg, which develops into a band, or stripe, of hard skin. Over time these linear bands may extend down into the underlying muscle and bone, causing awful deformities. Linear scleroderma is not pretty-looking, but it isn't life threatening. Linear and morphea sometimes occur together.

En coup de sabre (meaning "strike of the sword") scleroderma is another form of linear scleroderma. It is characterized by a linear stripe that affects the scalp and face. The depression in the forehead can look like a scar from dueling with swords. En coup de sabre can cause ocular, oral, and neurological complications, including seizures[2]

The en coup de sabre lesion may worsen, and it can cause atrophy of one side of the face (which is called hemifacial atrophy). If hemifacial atrophy occurs alone (in the absence of the typical lesion of en coupe de sabre on the forehead), then it is termed Parry-Rombergs Syndrome.

En Coup de Sabre
It is important to normalize chronic illness by seeking support and finding others like you. See, even this kangaroo has en coup!

In the deep subtypes of linear scleroderma with large involvement of a leg or an arm, severe contractures can develop with risk of permanent disability. In such patients an aggressive therapy is required. Though no controlled trials are available and only small case series are reported, corticosteroids (pulsed and oral) and methotrexate seem to be the more effective and safe therapy in severe localized scleroderma.[2]

Linear scleroderma tends to be chronic or progressive, and especially, en coup de sabre. Consulting a scleroderma expert center at the earliest possible stage is highly recommended.

Juvenile Systemic Sclerosis (jSSc)

Juvenile systemic sclerosis (jSSc) is a connective tissue disease involving the skin and underlying tissue and later affecting internal organs such as the lungs, gastrointestinal tract, kidneys and heart.

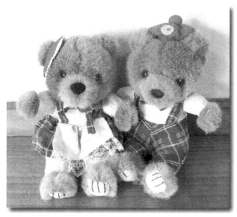

The development of the disease is the same as reported in *Chapter 1* for systemic sclerosis (SSc) in adulthood, however, the term juvenile systemic sclerosis (jSSc) is reserved for systemic scleroderma that onsets during childhood.

Like the adult version, juvenile systemic sclerosis is also subdivided into diffuse cutaneous systemic scleroderma (dSSc) or limited cutaneous systemic scleroderma (lSSc), according to the extent of skin involvement.

Juvenile systemic sclerosis (jSSc) occurs equally in boys and girls when the disease begins before age 8. After that age, it onsets predominantly in girls.

In juvenile systemic sclerosis (jSSc), both boys and girls are affected equally when the disease begins under 8 years of age. When onset begins after age 8, it seems to affect more girls than boys.

In children, the diffuse form accounts for about 25% of all jSSc cases.[4] Diffuse jSSc and limited jSSc are not easily distinguishable in children, and the prognosis is comparable in both forms. With any form of jSSc, the internal organs may be involved. Thus, there may be a wide variety of symptoms, and over time, serious damage to the affected organs can be life threatening.

Symptoms of Juvenile Systemic Sclerosis (jSSc)

The disease onset of juvenile systemic sclerosis (jSSc) is very gradual in most cases, so the diagnosis may be delayed by weeks to months due to the lack of specific symptoms.

A warm and tender swelling of the skin and underlying tissues involving face, hands, arms, toes and/or trunk may be the first noticeable symptom of the disease, long before skin tightening or hardening occurs.

The skin involvement in jSSc typically occurs symmetrically and often begins in the hands, making the fingers appear puffy. The skin does not change color (as it does in morphea) or develop linear indentations (as it does with linear scleroderma).

The usually slow progression of colorless skin changes makes it hard to reach the proper diagnosis. Often, many diseases are suggested at this point, and the child is referred to a dermatologist. When the initial treatment doesn't work and the skin hardening begins, the family usually seeks further help.

In this phase the skin becomes progressively harder, thin, and it adheres to the underlying tissues, making it difficult or impossible to pinch the skin. The hands, face and trunk may show impressive changes, with a typical symmetrical distribution.

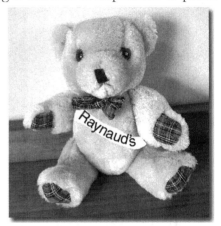

The fingers may become rigid and skin sores (known as digital ulcers) may develop, usually in the fingertips.

If the child's face is affected, it may become tighter, losing its natural wrinkles and expressiveness. The entire mouth may become smaller (which is called microstomia). Fine blood vessels may dilate on the face, causing painless "red dots" about the

Raynaud's makes colorful hands and feet! One or more fingers or toes may briefly turn white and/or blue and then, perhaps, red.

size of a pimple, or smaller, that are called telangiectasias.

Often children are not recognized as having scleroderma until they develop Raynaud's phenomenon. Raynaud's is often the initial symptom of juvenile systemic sclerosis (jSSc), beginning years before skin changes and other symptoms; however the majority of people with Raynaud's never develop scleroderma or other connective tissue diseases, so Raynaud's by itself is not ominous.

Raynaud's presents as a color change in one or more fingers or toes. The color changes may go from white (blanching) and/or blue (cyanosis) as blood supply is temporarily interrupted due to spasms of the blood vessels. As the circulation returns, the affected areas sometimes briefly turn pink or red (erythema). Raynaud's is more evident in the fingertips or toes, though it may occur anywhere, often on the tip of the nose or the ears.

During the course of the disease, symptoms related to internal organs may develop. Difficulty swallowing (dysphagia) affects almost one-fourth of children with juvenile systemic sclerosis (jSSc). It is caused by heartburn and esophageal dysmotility.

Small bowel involvement may cause abdominal pain, diarrhea, malabsorption, and slow growth. At onset, some children have major musculoskeletal symptoms with joint pain (arthralgia) and joint contractures, leading to the diagnosis of juvenile arthritis.

Heart and lung disease (cardiopulmonary) is usually absent at onset, but it eventually develops in many children with jSSc. This complication is the leading cause of death in those with diffuse jSSc, while kidney (renal) involvement is less common in children than in adults with systemic sclerosis (SSc).

Treatment of Juvenile Systemic Sclerosis (jSSc)

The best hope for these children is to be aggressively treated once their scleroderma has been recognized in order to prevent or slow the progress of internal organ involvement.

Since this is a rare and complex illness, children with juvenile systemic sclerosis (jSSc) should be under the care of an experienced juvenile scleroderma specialist. Scleroderma centers are best equipped to monitor closely for internal organ involvement and to provide advice on the latest treatments.

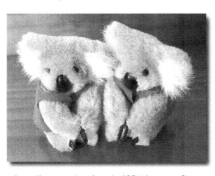

Juvenile systemic sclerosis (jSSc) is a rare disease which should be treated by scleroderma experts.

No uniformly effective therapy exists for either limited or diffuse juvenile systemic sclerosis (jSSc), and no treatment has proven to be effective in halting the disease progression.

Most of the treatment regimens have significant possible side effects, so the beneficial effect of several drugs must be carefully balanced with toxicity. Proper treatment for jSSc may require a series of drugs over time, or even a combination of agents. Fortunately, many treatments for symptoms of jSSc have been proven effective.

At onset, corticosteroids have shown to be effective in reducing muscle inflammation, fatigue, and pain. Some children have been treated with cyclosporine or methotrexate with beneficial effects, but larger studies are required to confirm such preliminary data.

Autologous hemopoietic stem cell transplantation, one of the most aggressive therapies, should be considered at disease onset before fibrosis has irreparably damaged the lungs, heart, and kidneys. However, owing to a high death rate (mortality) from this procedure, it is considered very cautiously.

Prognosis of Juvenile Systemic Sclerosis (jSSc)

New aggressive therapeutic approaches and continually improving treatments for symptoms herald a better long-term prognosis for both diffuse and limited juvenile systemic sclerosis (jSSc) than older literature suggests. A recent 19-year follow-up study found a 99% survival after one year of illness, and a 94% survival after 8 years of jSSc. Overall, outcomes are much better for jSSc than for adult-onset SSc.[4]

Conclusion

Children with scleroderma may benefit greatly from consultation with scleroderma experts, which can be found listed on the ISN website at www.sclero.org. As much as possible, children with scleroderma should be encouraged to live full and active lives.

Parents can make an enormous difference by helping their children develop positive attitudes and confidence regarding their unlimited ability to adjust to the varying effects of scleroderma on their health and appearance. Seeking and following expert care, as well as scleroderma and caregiver support and information, are the best measures for improving the lives of children who have scleroderma.

References

[1] Is Juvenile Localized Scleroderma really "LOCALIZED"? One fourth of JLS patients in this data series presented various kind of extra-cutaneous manifestations...These findings should change our clinical approach to this disease and underline the need for systemic immunosuppressive treatment for some patients. Francesco Zulian, R Russo, R Laxer, R Cuttica, G Espada, F Corona, M Mukamel, R Vesely, EM Nowakowska, J Chaitow, J Ros, MT Apaz, V Gerloni, B De Liphaus, S Nielsen, G Horneff, T Herlin, C Wouters, H Mazur-Zielinska, T Saurenmann, T Avcin, D Galic, G Martini, BH Athreya, for the Juvenile Scleroderma Working group of PRES. University of Padua, Padua, Italy. Arch Dermatol. 2005 Jul;141(7):847-52.

[2] Pulsed high-dose corticosteroids combined with low-dose methotrexate in severe localized scleroderma (LS). "These data suggest that pulsed high-dose corticosteroids combined with orally administered low-dose methotrexate therapy is beneficial and safe in the treatment of patients with LS. This treatment regimen should especially be considered for severe forms of LS in which conventional treatments have failed." Kreuter A, Gambichler T, Breuckmann F, Rotterdam S, Freitag M, Stuecker M, Hoffmann K, Altmeyer P.; Department of Dermatology and Allergology, Ruhr-University Bochum, Bochum, Germany. PubMed. Arch Dermatol. 2005 Jul;141(7):847-52.

[3] Localized scleroderma in adults and children. Clinical and laboratory investigations in 239 cases. Marzano AV, Menni S, Parodi A, Borghi A, Fuligni A, Fabbri P, Caputo R; Institute of Dermatological Sciences of the University of Milan and IRCCS Ospedale Maggiore of Milan, Italy; Eur J Dermatol. 2003 Mar-Apr;13(2):171-6.

[4] Juvenile Systemic Sclerosis: A Follow-up Study of Eight Patients. Szamosi S, Marodi L, Czirjak L, Ellenes Z, Szucs G. Third Department of Medicine, Division of Rheumatology, University of Debrecen Medical Center, Hungary. Ann N Y Acad Sci. 2005 Jun;1051:229-34.

[5] Localized scleroderma is an autoimmune disorder. Takehara K, Sato S.; Department of Dermatology, Kanazawa University Graduate School of Medical Sciences, Kanazawa, Japan. Rheumatology (Oxford). 2005 Mar;44(3):274-9.

Angela
Louisiana, USA

I have a sixteen-year-old daughter who was diagnosed with linear scleroderma twelve years ago. It began on her hip and spread to her lower limbs. Now she has a great deal of atrophy in one leg and foot.

She has gone through two surgeries to straighten toes and stretch the heel cord. She is an active teenager and she plays basketball and jogs occasionally.

However, she now deals with a great deal of pain when her leg goes into spasms. These usually occur in the evening while at rest, but may happen anytime and are quite painful.

We are in search of others who might share this problem and also some who may have solutions to help deal with the pain.

Update – June 2003

My daughter is now seventeen and in addition to her sport activities and schooling she maintains a waitress job.

She still has painful leg spasms but sometimes at bedtime she will take medicine for it, and that seems to help her to rest for the rest of the night, but even that takes awhile to work.

I would like to offer a word of encouragement for others who share any painful disorder. Since my child has had this condition since the age of four, we have had several opportunities to pray over her. I can honestly say that even though her body is not whole, her spirituality certainly is.

In spite of all the physical and emotional pain that scleroderma has brought her, she is more whole because of it. Yet, as a mother who still witnesses her child in much physical pain, I am constantly seeking others to offer solutions that may help her.

◆❖◆

Annabella
Colorado, USA

A mother's intuition never fails. When I first noticed the marks on my little girl's left thigh during bath time last summer, I got a sick feeling in my stomach. Right away I showed the marks to my husband and said that I thought it was morphea. I am not a medical professional. I just had a feeling about it because my sixteen-year-old niece has had morphea on her face since she was five, so I was already familiar with what it may look like.

Even after two doctors misdiagnosed the marks, I still insisted on another opinion and that brought me to a dermatologist who agreed with my original gut feeling. Since August 2002 my little four-year-old angel has had marks appear all over; one on her right butt cheek, one on her lower back, two on her torso, two on her foot, and the small marks on her thigh have taken over the entire length of her leg in a matter of months.

We are at a crossroads now. Do we give her drugs or continue the ultraviolet UVA-1 light therapy? The light therapy has softened up the spots remarkably but I just noticed some new growth on her other leg. Do we try drugs at such a tender age?

Update – May 2003

"Mommy it hurts," she cries.

I am a desperate mother in a frantic search for stories of other parents who have children who suffer from morphea.

Another spot has appeared. When will it end? "Mommy it hurts" keeps ringing in my ears at bedtime and I cannot stand the emotional heartache any longer.

Gabrialla was diagnosed back in August 2002, and has seven new growths since then. The most serious one covers her entire left leg. We are afraid it will hinder the growth in that leg, her mobility, and scar it for life.

She is at such a tender age so we do not know if we should try drugs. We currently have her on UVA-1 light therapy and it is softening up the skin, but we want to know if drugs like methotrexate can stop new growths from forming?

◆❖◆

Cindy Fuchs-Morrissey
Missouri, USA

My name is Cindy Fuchs-Morrissey from Macon, Missouri. Our daughter Hilary, has scleroderma in the form of progressive systemic sclerosis. She turned thirteen several days ago and will be in eighth grade for the 2003-2004 school year.

Hilary has an aggressive form of scleroderma with swallowing problems, bowel problems, fatigue, severe joint and bone pain, fevers for no reason, allergies, and acral bone dysplasia of the hands and feet. Her hands and feet are the size of an eleven to fifteen month old child. They have fused and will not grow much larger.

She often has extreme joint and bone pain in her tiny hands, knees, feet and ankles, elbows and shoulders. Her shoulders are popping out like she is coming unglued. She says this is very painful. Some days she feels like a very stiff old lady. She wears hand splints at night, and uses a wheelchair to help reduce the pain of walking on her tiny infant feet. The wheelchair has been extremely helpful in aiding a better quality of life for her.

Hilary has had an esophageal motility test which was abnormal with decreased lower esophageal sphincter pressure and slightly decreased lower peristalsis in the distal esophagus. I really did not need this test to tell me she had a problem swallowing, but I decided to have it done only so the doctors would know that I was telling them the truth. We will never allow Hilary to go through another esophageal motility test, as we feel she is suffering enough without more tests being run.

Hilary's swallowing problem has gotten worse, which scares her. It waxes and wanes like the joint and bone pain, swelling, and other symptoms. She is also having a very bad bowel problem, which is frustrating.

In November 2001, Hilary was found to have an insulin resistance problem that caused acanthosis nigricans (AN), which is black skin on top of her scleroderma shiny, varnished skin. For the AN, Hilary used medicinal creams that burned her skin. The AN just comes back. It is very difficult to clean the black skin under her armpits. Her neck looks better now, but the black skin is returning again.

Somebody is always making a comment that she needs to clean her neck as it can become very dark and dirty looking. But her neck is very clean! If the general public was better informed and educated about these types of health problems and really knew what this little girl is going through they would not make such comments.

Hilary also has had seven of her toenails removed as they were very deformed and causing her great pain. This surgery has helped Hilary's quality of life as she does not have to deal with the extremely painful, deformed toenails anymore. She did heal, but healed slowly as she does not heal normally. In July 2003, she will be having her three remaining toenails removed. She is looking forward to this so that she will not have to experience the pain that the toenails have caused in the past.

She was on a glucocorticoid for a short time when she was younger which made her gain weight and made her less tired, but made her very crabby! But it did not help her tissues at all. We have opted against other medical treatments and testing at this time. We have just decided to allow nature to runs its course for now, and Hilary is okay with this. We felt this would give her some quality of life.

I believe that Hilary's health problems are a result of my having silicone gel breast implants. In the winter of 1992, I requested a copy of my operation records. As I read through them, I felt I was opening a Pandora's Box.

I turned eighteen in November 1976, and the next week I opted for silicone gel breast implant surgery to correct a congenital deformity of the chest wall (not for larger breasts.) This surgery was a birthday present from my mom and dad, a birthday present I would never forget!

Soon after the surgery, I started having a lot of hair loss. I felt like I had the flu and I was feeling a lot of fatigue and some joint pain. The first Christmas after my implants, I had an allergy to the Christmas tree, of all things. I had never before had any health problems or allergies.

My health concerns slowly worsened. In July 1978, I had to have the 1976 implants replaced. They were now rock hard and extremely painful. Unfortunately, both implants had ruptured, but oddly my plastic surgeon never told me or my parents about it. We found out about this in the early 1990s when I requested my medical records.

During the 1978 surgery, the surgeon dropped a bovie (a digital electro surgical generator) on my stomach and breast, and this left scars. Of course, the doctor had to tell us about that, as the scars could be seen.

In the winter of 1978, I had a close capsule release and an injection of trigger pain point anterior axillary line. With that procedure I had a severe adverse reaction to the medication used to sedate me.

In January 1980, my doctor replaced my left side implant, which was my problem side, with a lumen gel/saline breast implant. They did an open capsular release of the left breast with decortication of scar and fibrous capsule and reconstruction of congenital asymmetry with another silicone implant.

I was under the impression that breast implants would last a lifetime and I thought they had been fully investigated and were considered safe for any offspring and with breastfeeding. But I have since found that breast implants were not fully investigated with the offspring, or with breastfeeding.

I have learned that Hilary's health problems are probably the result of a silicone gel breast implant birth defect. My maternal grandmother had very deforming rheumatoid arthritis, and died from multiple myeloma. My mom died from multiple myeloma in June 1994.

I have multiple sclerosis (MS), elevated IgM antibodies, allergies, asthma, a poorly defined connective tissue problem, and more. What has happened in our family is that a genetically offending trigger has elevated our disease risk by affecting the variants of certain key genes.

We were HLA-typed at Thomas Jefferson University in 1998 in fetal cells in scleroderma study, as I personally questioned the microchimerism and chimerism with silicone Gel breast implants and the variants of certain key genes that could not embrace genetically offending triggers.

Hilary is registered with the Scleroderma Family Registry and DNA Repository in Houston, and the National Registry for Childhood Onset Scleroderma in Pittsburgh and in other more recent studies in molecular genetics.

In May 2003, Hilary had sixteen inches of her very long hair cut and donated to Wigs for Kids, an organization that makes wigs for children who have lost their hair due to chemotherapy treatments, burns or alopecia. So far she has had thirty-five inches cut and donated to Wigs for Kids.

Hilary's hair donation was my Mother's Day present. She wanted to give my hands a vacation from doing her hair every day as my MS has gotten worse. She loves to make others happy with her hair donations, and is hoping to grow it out again to donate it for a third time in high school.

There is so much more to my story. Someone could write a book about it, as I am tired of this mess.

◆ ❖ ◆

Debra Reynolds
Australia

Emma was just eighteen months old when a particular rash started on her torso. We took her to our general practitioner and he said it was just a rash.

Then I noticed a 'dinting' affect on Em's shins. After our pediatrician saw her, he sent us to our major hospital that is six hours from our home. All we were told was that Em had linear scleroderma. From there we read everything we could. This was not good. Through what we learned then, we thought she only had a short time to live, since we thought all forms of scleroderma were similar.

Well, here we are and Emma is now thirteen years old. She has gone through a lot, but she has never asked, "Why me?" Emma is the most courageous person I know. She did not have a normal childhood as she was always with doctors and nurses. They even call her 'the forty-year-old midget.'

Recently the specialist told us that her disease is burnt out, as Em has had no more new sites. So now we are going to fix what the disease has damaged. We are looking at skin grafts, collagen injections and whatever else is needed. Emma is not taking any medication now. Apart from the occasional emotional fit, she is doing great.

I now am beginning to research this disease. I did not think many people had scleroderma, but I now am finding and talking to lots of people with the same thing. It is so good to have support and be able to ask questions and have them answered. Now I can explain to Emma what is going on.

All in all, I think I have the most incredible daughter and hope that other people respect and support their loved ones with this disease.

◆❖◆

Helen
Poland

We used to live in New York, and when my daughter was four, when I discovered a small spot on her left foot. I did not want to despair, but after awhile I took her to my dermatologist, and he gave the right diagnosis of morphea.

I did not know anything about morphea in the beginning, so I went on the Internet and then cried for a few days. At the same time I started to look for a doctor. Even though I was living in a big city it was not easy to find the right one.

Finally, I found one of the best known morphea doctors and my daughter started her treatment. The doctor gave her a medication. She took it for almost two years, but it did not make any changes or improvements. Then I went to another doctor, and he advised me to drop all medication and just check her every six months.

When Sonia was seven, we decided to go back to Europe, and I tried to find a doctor over here. We went to Poland and started her treatment there. I cannot say that it is better here, but we receive different treatment. It has not helped so far, but I am hoping that finally something will start working.

In the meantime, the disease has spread on her whole left leg, and some spots have appeared on her right leg and a few spots on her belly. I tried almost everything, including unconventional medicine, but I still have the feeling that I missed something. I know there has to be some medication or treatment that can help.

Linda Egginger
Minnesota, USA

My daughter Kate, was diagnosed with morphea in May 2002. She is nine years old now.

Last summer I noticed what I thought was a really big bruise on the right side of her stomach. I asked her if she had been hit by anything that she could remember and she said no. She is a very active child so I did not think any more about it.

Five weeks later I noticed that the bruise was still there so we went to a pediatrician who referred us to a dermatologist. The dermatologist basically said that it was no big deal and could not remember the name of what he thought it was. I was not happy with this response so we went to another dermatologist who looked her over with a black light so he could see if there were more spots forming under her skin. He got out all his medical books and showed us pictures and said that he wanted to see her whenever she got a new spot.

About a month went by and we did notice more. She now had two on the right side of her back by her shoulder blades and another one starting on her right arm. She had also developed a line starting at her hairline just to the right of her nose and going down to the top of her nose. So we went back to the doctor. He said that this was called en coupe de sabre.

Everything was going fine and she did not hurt anywhere, but some kids at school were starting to notice her forehead and making jokes about it. We went back to the dermatologist yesterday and he came in the room, looked at her and said, "We need to get her to a rheumatologist right away." That really scared me. He seemed very concerned because she had developed another spot on her forehead.

I am very nervous about this rheumatologist appointment that we have on January 15th. I do not want her to be poked and prodded if nothing is going to help. I guess I do not know what to expect. I know that there is no cure for what she has and I think that Kate and my husband and I have adjusted to that. I guess I will find out what happens next. Kate has been reading some of the stories and I think that they are helping her to realize that she is not the only person who has this. I will keep you posted on what the doctor says at the next visit. Thanks for reading my story. It helps to share it. I am still scared, but hopeful.

Update – January 2003

We had our first rheumatologist appointment on Wednesday. The doctor talked to us for almost three hours. She explained everything to Kate. The doctor said that if Kate had another type of localized scleroderma, she probably would not treat her at all and just let the disease run its course. But she said that the line on Kate's forehead could move down her face or further into her head and cause bone deformities. So she prescribed prednisone and methotrexate. She said that Kate might get puffy from the steroids and that the methotrexate could make her sick to her stomach. She also said that Kate's appetite would increase so we will have to watch what she eats. This is exactly the kind of thing that I did not want to happen! I do not want Kate to become a different person because of this disease! But what are my options? Either we just wait to see if it spreads or we could try to put a stop to it.

I am very sad about this whole thing, I just about cry every time I give her the medication.

Update – March 2003

We had a rheumatologist appointment last Wednesday and we can start to lower her dosage of the prednisone finally.

She has gained eleven pounds and is constantly harassed at school because she is fat. She comes home just about every day and cries. She does not want to tell them why she has gained weight because then she thinks she will have to explain the whole disease and they would tease her even more if they knew about her spots.

I hope that when she is off this medication she will lose the weight that she has gained. It would make her feel better. She is a very beautiful girl who never says anything bad about anyone and she does not deserve this.

Anyway, she has had no more spots show up that we know of so that is one good thing. The doctor has increased her dosage of methotrexate and we go back to see her in a month.

Update – August 2003

Kate is doing much better. She is off the prednisone and has lost all the weight that she gained while she was on it. She is still on the methotrexate. She takes it once a week. Her lesions are barely visible now and the en coupe de saber is less noticeable. People who have not seen her in a while do not even notice it.

I am not sure that if the morphea flares up again that I would do the steroid again. It was very hard on her but it seemed to work. Her rheumatologist said that she may be on the methotrexate for a year or longer depending on how she tolerates it, but so far she is doing well. Her doctor appointments are down to once every three months. Her next one is in September. After that if no more lesions develop her next appointment will be in six months.

I am hoping that the worst is behind her and that it does not flare up again.

Update – March 2004

Kate is doing much better. The lesions on her back are barely visible. The large one on her stomach is still there, but it is just indented, and no longer discolored. Her forehead scar is also doing better. It has not grown in length, width, or depth. She is still on the methotrexate and could be on it for up to five years, but she seems to be tolerating it okay.

She is at a different school now and no one there knows anything about her disease unless she wants them to. She has made some very good friends and is doing quite well. This disease has taken a little bit of her spark away, but I think she will be okay. It seems to have just become part of her now.

I want to thank everyone who has written me. It really helps. If I can help you in any way, please do not hesitate to write to me.

❖

Sharon Hill
Australia

My name is Shaz and my seven-year-old son has had morphea since he was five. Recently he developed skin tightening on his hands, similar to limited scleroderma, and it has spread quite rapidly.

It has been very hard for us to find much information on his condition and I am asking for anyone's help on this. He has morphea on his chest, shoulders, arms and hands.

When we were first told about the morphea we thought he would have a few spots and nothing else major would come of it. Now we have been told he could have some serious problems.

We have an appointment with a rheumatologist tomorrow morning and we are very anxious to find out more information about what we can do to help our son cope with this. I am so glad I found this web site as now I do not feel so alone on this scary journey that we have been forced to take.

CHAPTER 6

Localized Scleroderma
Linear and Morphea

I hope there are people who read this story before they jump to the wrong conclusions like I did

—Joyce Romkes

Cedric Goliath
Linear Scleroderma
South Africa

I have been reasonably healthy, am married and have two healthy boys. I was particularly worried about some things, and as a result I experienced terrible stomach cramps and excruciating migraines. I visited my local general practitioner (GP) for these ailments and was referred to a hospital. A sample of my stools was taken but the results showed nothing. I was told to stay away from foods like coffee and chocolate to ease my migraines.

I became aware of a small brown spot just above my right eye and gradually this patch became bigger and darker. People asked me if I had walked into a door because by this time an indent started to appear in exactly the same place as the brown patch. During this time I was experiencing so much stress that I could have given up on life. I was twenty-nine years of age.

More dark spots appeared behind my neck, over my body, and on my arms. I was referred to the dermatology department of the hospital where a biopsy was performed. The professor/doctor diagnosed me with linear scleroderma combined with en coup de sabre. According to her this is very rare in South Africa. She also confirmed that it is not systemic and thus not life threatening. Phew, what a relief!

I provided my local general practitioner (GP), Doctor Tripp, with current information of this condition from the Internet. He was very pleased to receive this and after scrutinizing it, he prompted me to try using sun block on the patch. I tried this but with no change.

My eldest son is suffering with eczema and is using a special ointment for it. Feeling desperate, I tried this ointment and experienced a funny sensation on my linear patch and indentation. Somehow the patch started to fade but small white spots started to appear in the left corner of my right eye. I immediately stopped with the ointment and instead used Vitamin E cream. What a difference.

The patch is very noticeably fading. At times when I feel stressed out, I get this funny sensation that is also abating. Maybe I am onto something good. I feel healthier and more positive, although the condition has never really troubled me. The only down side to this was that I knew it was there and became more aware of it when people stared at it.

I am still continuing to use the cream, hoping that the spots will disappear completely. I was told the en coup de sabre could be corrected with a collagen injection, but this is very expensive in South Africa.

Now I am happily married, with three healthy happy boys, and financially secure. I praise God every day of my life that I have the time to spend with my family, friends and contemporaries.

This is my life.

Joyce Romkes
Linear Scleroderma
Holland

When I was fifteen years old, somebody at school pointed out to me the fact that there was a white spot in the middle of my forehead, just below the hairline. I thought it was nothing, but then more people started to notice. I realized that this spot was actually growing. So I decided to go see my doctor, and he measured the spot. He told me to come back next week to see if it was actually growing like I thought it was.

The next week the spot was three times bigger! My doctor sent me to a dermatologist, and the dermatologist took two skin samples.

When I went back two weeks later, the dermatologist told me he was not sure what the spot was. He then let about six other doctors come in and look at me. Then the doctors debated for about a half hour and they told me it was scleroderma en coup de sabre. Unfortunately, they did not know anything about it, so I looked it up on the Internet. Not a good thing to do, especially not when the first stories you get to read are the ones about diffuse scleroderma. I totally panicked.

Luckily, a scleroderma group sent me a booklet that explained my situation. I was so relieved.

I am twenty-two now, and the scleroderma is still there. I have a white stripe dividing my forehead into two parts, and I think there might be something growing next to it on the right side.

I hope there are people who read this story before they jump to the wrong conclusions like I did!

I want to thank everyone who has worked on making information about scleroderma available.

Leon Schelfhout
Linear Scleroderma
The Netherlands

This story was translated into English by Ans Mens. The original story is in Chapter 11.

They discovered two spots on my left forearm when I was five years old. Our family doctor sent me to a dermatologist, who could make nothing of it, so they sent me to a neurologist.

The neurologist did two things: a spinal tap and a penicillin cure by needle. This I do not forget my entire life. He also wanted to put "no diagnosis." This took place in 1962-63.

I was referred to a dermatologist in the academic hospital in Leiden. This was a long voyage, since we lived in Zeeuws-Vlaanderen (which was far south of Leiden) and traveling was not well-regulated then.

In the AZL they did a lot of research, one which involved removing a bit of skin/tissue. I was sent home with an ointment that I had to put on my arm each evening before sleeping with my arm packed in plastic, which I did for many years.

In the meantime I detected that I could not bend my left wrist and my left arm was less developed than the other. In the AZL, I was referred to an orthopaedic surgeon. In my eleventh year my arm was operated on, to see how it looked inside. There was a lot of connective tissue in the muscles and tendons.

In that time the electromyogram (EMG) was discovered, so I also experienced that. When I was twelve and older, my visits to the hospital were as an out patient.

The diagnosis of my spot was called dermasclerose, but they could not do anything for it. For years I have had less functioning in my left arm and hand, and I have learned to live with it.

In my twenties, I saw the hospital from inside again—as a male nurse! I knew my limitations, so I was able to function well.

Then I had more trouble with my wrist, it was leaning backwards. In my twenty-fifth year, an orthopaedic surgeon operated on my wrist. He tried to extend the tendons by splitting them.

In the preliminary investigation for that surgery, I was examined by a professor of dermatology in the Academic Hospital Nijmegen. Then I heard for the first time the definitive diagnosis, dermasclerose linear, and learned that it is a childhood disease, but has no cure.

Unfortunately, the operation did not yield the desired result. I still have limitations. I am no longer a nurse; I am now a logistics co-worker.

At forty-seven, I am once again confronted with this illness. I sat behind the computer every day and performed tasks for one and a half years with the burden of a painful left hand, especially the fingers, which feel like a hundred needle sticks.

My general practitioner said this is repetitive strain injury (RSI) and referred me through to a business physician. I told him my previous history and he came to the same conclusion. He did not know about scleroderma, but he sought information on it. Long live the Internet! His diagnosis is clear: my scleroderma follows me again!

Lisa Kate McGowan
Linear Scleroderma
Australia

I was diagnosed with linear scleroderma when I was eighteen. It changed my life because it affected my left arm by leaving a big shiny scar on it.

People always asked me what happened. They asked if I had been hit (as it looked like a bruise) or if I had been burnt. I told them the truth when I first was diagnosed, but then it became embarrassing as people thought it was contagious (which it isn't). So I made up a story about how a pot of boiling water fell on my arm when I was little. People seem satisfied with that.

The pain in my left arm was very hard to describe as it hurt from the inside rather than on the surface. But on the outside it would sometimes become very itchy and inflamed. My doctor prescribed methotrexate, which I took on a weekly basis. I was not one of the lucky ones with this medication as I became very ill and sick all the time. It lowered my immunity so I picked up every bug that went around.

I lost over six kilos (about thirteen pounds) in a month, and weighed only forty-eight kilos (about one hundred and five pounds). I am one hundred and seventy-four centimeters (about five feet and seven inches) tall. People would often comment on my weight and refer to me as anorexic. I was too embarrassed to tell them that I was ill and on very strong medication.

My feet were always cold and sometimes they would appear almost black in color. When I got bruises on my leg, they would stay there for months. My linear-affected arm was much smaller than my other arm, and I became very self-conscious when wearing singlets (tank tops) or tee shirts.

My health was so bad that if I had a late night, by the next morning I would have an infected throat or a bad cold which would eventually turn into the flu. I was always on antibiotics and trying new sorts of medicines to help me cope with the methotrexate, but generally, I had to cope with the nausea and side effects twenty-four hours a day.

When my doctor told me that I was going into remission, I was over the moon. My whole family was happy. But less than six months later, I was told that it was spreading again.

I continued with life as normally as I could, trying to build up my immune system. I found that if I cut the circulation off in my arm with a watch or carrying a bag, my arm would flare up and become very itchy. My skin looked like I had lots of red lumps on it. My condition was more annoying than anything, but the medication that was used to treat my disease was the main thing that I could not cope with.

Now I am twenty-one and I have been off my medication for over a year. I have been in remission for the same amount of time. I have to have checkups regularly to monitor any changes that may occur, but other than that, my life is back to normal. My immune system is a lot better now, but I have to be careful not to get sick as a simple cold still turns into a very bad flu.

My main concern these days is my legs and feet. They are always stone cold due to bad circulation, and if I ever get a cut or a bruise on my legs, it takes months for it to heal.

The scar on my arm still bothers me, but I am very lucky that that is all I have. Others have the scar on their face or other parts of their bodies.

I would love to speak to anyone who has a condition that is similar to mine. None of my friends or family really understands the physical and emotional effect that this has had on me. I never appreciated my health until this. I would love to be completely healthy.

Vanessa Betancourt
Linear Scleroderma
California, USA

I only lived four years of my life like a healthy, normal-looking kid.

My linear scleroderma started out like a big, long bruise on my forehead. My family was not very worried about it, as they thought I had just fallen and bumped my head. But the bruise did not go away and over the next few weeks it changed from a light pink to a purple.

Mom finally took me to the doctor who referred me to a dermatologist. The dermatologist said it was a reaction to the sun and gave me medication to put on my forehead every time I went out into the sun.

My mom knew it was not just a reaction, she knew it was worse, so I was taken to countless doctors and specialists for a diagnosis. Finally we got the news we had waited for so long: Linear Scleroderma.

My older sister found a way to cover up the nasty disease on my forehead. Bangs! It was a great idea! She gave me bangs when I was in kindergarten and I have had them ever since, twelve years later.

Growing up was hard. The right side of my face began to get disfigured. I was teased alot in elementary and middle school. Boys did not like me and people judged me because of the way I looked. It was really hard. Sometimes I did not feel like going to school because I knew someone would push my buttons.

Then began the best years of my life: high school! I have more friends and even an occasional boyfriend here and there. I even have a great one right now. He is the only guy I have told about my illness. I am too ashamed and embarrassed to tell anyone else.

My doctors say I could get corrective surgery to make me look like everyone else. I am debating if I should or not. If I do, then I will get it when I graduate from high school next year.

I have learned to live with the way I look. I cannot kick myself in the butt because of it. It is just the way my life happened.

Update – October 2004

I have gotten engaged, graduated high school, and found a job as a Certified Nurse Assistant (CNA). Plans for our wedding are still far away. We are hoping to get married in two to three years.

As for reconstructive surgery, I have decided against it. I have seen how it is done. I was really grossed out by it, and let me just say it is not my cup of tea! They said I would even have my mouth wired shut for a month. With my appetite, I would not last even for a couple days!

Alessandra Brustolon
Morphea
Italy

This story was translated from Italian to English by Kevin Howell. He is a Clinical Scientist for Professor Carol Black at the Royal Free Hospital in London. The Italian version of this story is in Chapter 10.

I am Alessandra, I am forty years old, and about a year and a half ago I was diagnosed with morphea.

I have patches on only the right side of my body: the back of the thigh, the hip, and in the groin area. My patches are reddish-brown but the skin is not hardened. It started out with a strong tingling (especially on the leg), but I have never had any pain. Lately the patch in the groin area has spread, despite the doctors at San Lazzaro Hospital seeing under the microscope that the disease is in a regressive phase.

Cindy
Morphea
Missouri, USA

I am thirty-three and I have morphea, which is a form of localized scleroderma.

I only recently learned that morphea is the name of the disease that has bothered me since the age of six. Way back then, my mother took me to the doctor and was simply told that I had a childhood skin disorder.

I have several scars from the affected areas that I had as a child. They began as small and slightly discolored round patches. They all turned white, hard and scaly. It took at least ten years for them to fade and turn into slightly depressed, darkened skin. They resemble a scar from a burn.

For more than a decade I had no new patches. What bothers me now are that I have new white spots on my right breast, and one of them is growing much faster and larger than any of the marks I had as a child.

I also suffer from joint pain, headaches, and lack of energy. I have not had any blood work or biopsies yet. My dermatologist is using a topical steroid cream to control the spreading, and he has advised me to see a rheumatologist.

Connie
Morphea
Canada

At age sixteen I developed what I thought were bruises on the biceps of both arms; two spots, same size and shape and everything, on both arms. I assumed they were bruises from carrying boxes, but they never went away. Then more came, and they were all symmetrical.

My first dermatologist diagnosed me with morphea. He said it was similar to scleroderma but not as bad, I had nothing to worry about, and it would go away on its own.

This scared me to death because my aunt has scleroderma and was not (and still is not) doing well. So I went to see another doctor who took a biopsy and told me I had morphea and lichen sclerosus et atrophicus. All my research afterward seemed to say that lichen sclerosus primarily affected the genitals, and I had none of those symptoms.

Then at about age eighteen I developed a single spot, the first one that did not come with a twin. This spot became itchy and it was smoother than the rest of my back. It was also much larger than any of my other spots, about the size of my hand spread out. I had given up on trying to find out about the disease so I left the spot alone and it hardened and became shiny.

At about age twenty-two I saw yet another dermatologist who said the disease must be burnt out because no new spots had developed in the last four years. And since the spot on my back was not really bothering me, I should just go home and not worry about it. So that is what I have done.

In the last two years, a few new spots have developed on my breasts and hips. I also had a seizure two years ago that was followed by an MRI which showed what was only explained to me as being a white dot. Nobody seems to give me a straight answer, no matter how many questions I ask. I am confused by the Internet information, because I cannot figure out which type of scleroderma I have, although I am convinced that it is not lichen sclerosis et atrophicus.

If the disease burns out, can it recur? Does stress affect the disease? I have also found research suggesting a connection between morphea and ankylosing spondilitis, which my father has. In all, I will be twenty-nine soon, which will make it thirteen years with no answers.

◆❖◆

Crystal
Morphea
Canada

I am thirty years old and I have morphea. I was diagnosed with it when I was ten. It started on my stomach and then spread to my legs.

One day when I was at school I was called to the office and asked if my parents were abusive. I was mortified. That was the last time I wore shorts for a long time.

My mother took me to a skin specialist and all I remember was that this could spread all over and there is no cure. I left the doctor's office in tears. My mother told me to stop my crying as I was not dying.

I realized over the years that my skin would get very itchy when the morphea was active. I have morphea on my back, over most of my legs, and on my arm.

I felt like a freak growing up and I felt so alone. Morphea limited my social life as I would never allow anyone to see it unless they were close friends. I was unable to keep a relationship with a man as I could not bear being humiliated if my little secret got out.

It was not until I was twenty-seven that I finally found someone who would not let me push him away, as he loved me. I thank God for him. We recently created a miracle, our son.

This is something I never thought I would ever have. I still am reluctant to wear shorts, but in time I hope that I will feel strong enough to deal with the ignorant people who have no idea how much a snicker, a stare, or a rude question can hurt someone's feelings.

Ell
Morphea
England

When I was seventeen I got three ridged circular marks on my arm, near the wrist. The marks were red, going pink, then lilac and white in the center. They eventually went away after about a year. My doctor could not diagnose it.

At twenty-one it is back on the same arm, only one mark this time, but bigger. It starts out solid, like eczema, and then spreads out into a circle, until it fades and leaves a slight shadow, which fades to nothing. I asked my present doctor what it could be, after explaining that my father has been a sufferer of morphea all his life and that another relative of ours also has morphea. The doctor looked up the symptoms on the Internet and told me it was probably morphea. If it had not been for my dad I would still be uncertain as to what the marks were.

I am very scared though, as I have heard and read so many worrisome things about morphea. I have not seen a dermatologist and my doctor knows nothing about the condition.

I do not know if it will get worse, what type it could be or if I can give it to any children I may have in the future.

I get severe pain in the wrist where the morphea comes up and have problems with my joints. I would like to know if it is linked and where I should go for help. I do not know if it will spread or come up in other places or if it affects other areas of health.

I did not know anyone else had morphea outside my family, so it is a relief to know I can ask for help from people who understand.

I am thankful I now know what it is and that it is still not very serious.

◆❖◆

Faye Watson
Morphea
Australia

My name is Faye, and I am Scottish. When I was six or seven, I developed what looked like a bruise on the front of my left thigh. It started as a small purplish spot. My mother was very worried when it did not go away, so I was taken back and forth to the hospital.

Many doctors scratched their head as no one seemed to know what this strange thing was. "Could it be leprosy?" I was asked. "Have you any pain?" "No," I replied. And because I had no problems walking they lost interest. I was later told it was a rare skin condition called morphea, and from then on I was left in the dark.

My mum thinks that I was knocked hard on my leg while out playing, and that is what caused it.

The bruise grew to full size in my teenage years and has now, thankfully, stopped growing. It is about seven inches long and four inches wide. It is shaped like a picture of a rabbit, of all things!

I have lost some of my thigh muscle as it has grown, but I am in perfect health, for which I am grateful! It does not stop me from doing anything at all. I can walk, run, swim and ski. But sometimes at night I get aching pain. I worry about people staring at me when I am in my swimsuit, but that is no big deal. I get very tired and stressed easily, which I have been learning to control over the years.

I am now twenty-nine, living in Sydney, Australia, and getting married in February, so I have lots to look forward to!

❖ ❖ ❖

Lisa Dunnington
Morphea
England, UK

I will be thirty-five in a few months, and I am happily married with a ten year old healthy daughter. I have had morphea scleroderma for twenty-eight years.

I first noticed it when I was seven years old. It started as a dry patch of skin on my right arm. It took three years before I was diagnosed. I was put through a series of very unpleasant tests, and all the while it was spreading through my body. The doctors insisted that it would burn itself out eventually, but it did not.

It spread very quickly into my right hand, leaving it bony and deformed. I was about eleven and terribly frightened as I thought it would keep spreading and I would never be able to go outside again and be a normal child.

My mum and dad were desperate for help and tried to find a solution through church, hypnosis, and spiritual healing. The last two I did not bother with. I wanted to believe the doctors.

Now I am facing the prospect of losing my left hand to this disease. I am scared and I feel unable to cope at times. My hands feel frozen and painful and I dread winter. I go to occupational therapy when it gets really bad. The hot wax machine gives me a little relief, and I have also tried those thermal hand warmers that you just shake.

I am not sure if I am just more sensitive than some, but I have had a lot of pain with this. I really sympathize with everybody who is living with this.

◆❖◆

Patricia M.
Morphea
Virginia, USA

In 1980 when I was pregnant with my first child, I was surprised one day to wake up and look at my breasts, which looked as if they were on fire.

I was very concerned so I went to my obstetrician and he was just as surprised as I was. He sent me to a dermatologist who did a biopsy on my breast. When I went back for the results he told me I had morphea. I had no idea what it was so I asked him to explain. He told me it was a form of arthritis. He gave me some type of cream to apply to my breasts.

He said it would be a good idea for me not to breastfeed, since he didn't know for sure if it would be a problem or not. I went through the next eighteen years not knowing any more than that. I would mention this on occasion to several doctors but they had never heard of morphea, or so they said.

My sister was diagnosed with scleroderma about two months ago after years of problems, and we were looking up on the Internet information for her when I saw morphea. I still don't understand it, but at least I know I didn't dream this up. Now I still don't know if I should try to find out anything more about it or not, but at least I know this was real.

Rodolfo E. Claudet
Morphea
Peru

This story was translated from Spanish to English by Edwin Lamoli-Torres, who is a retired professor from the University of Puerto Rico at Mayaguez. The Spanish version of this story is in Chapter 9.

Hi! My name is Rodolfo. A year ago, I was diagnosed with localized scleroderma (morphea). I received assistance from a doctor here in Peru, but without any motive that I can understand, the treatment was discontinued. I have blemishes on my back and I have noticed that others are beginning to show where others had already appeared.

I would like to hear your advice and suggestions.

PART 3

Autoimmune and Overlap

CHAPTER 7

Autoimmune Stories

*I have learned to take control,
and I am not afraid anymore.*
—Patty Sandoval Sralla

Robin Hill
End Stage Renal Disease (ESRD)
Nevada, USA

I have been going through the pain of kidney failure for four years now. In this essay I will tell you my story of all I went through with this disease; all the surgeries I had to have, all the doctors I now have to keep up with, and all the pain I had to deal with. I hope by reading this you will come to understand what a person deals with when having to go through kidney failure.

It all started on October 30, 2000. I was sent into the lab for a routine blood test. After I had my blood drawn that day, all we were waiting for was the results. The next day, Halloween to be exact, the lab called. The nurse that had called me told me I was in renal failure. I was terrified. I had no idea what renal failure was, or what it was affecting. All I knew was I had to get to the emergency room (ER) and fast.

I quickly called my mom, who called her supervisor so she could get off work to pick me up. Within fifteen minutes she had come to take me to the ER. By this time, I was so weak I could barely walk down the stairs to get to the car. The disease was hitting me fast and hard.

When we arrived at the ER, I had to sit and wait to be admitted. After about twenty minutes I was seen by a doctor and was prepped for immediate perma-cath surgery. A perma-cath is a tube that the doctors put up into your jugular vein so dialysis can be done. As soon as I was out of surgery, I was on dialysis. The first three days I was in the intensive care unit because my condition was so severe. The doctors told my mother that if I had gotten to the ER any later I would have been dead.

As time went by I started to get better. I spent a total of two weeks in the hospital, but it was not the last stay I would have. Having routine dialysis treatments and checkups I was starting to feel myself again. But in the back of my mind I knew I would never be the real me again. I knew there would be many things in my life I would have to watch out for. I would realize this as the next four years went by.

There are three different ways to do dialysis. I have tried them all. The first I tried was hemodialysis. This is where you are hooked up to a machine and have to sit in a chair for four hours. While you sit in the chair the machine cleanses your blood. This happens by either a tube in the forearm or a tube up in the jugular vein in the neck. I tried this type of dialysis for a year. I have had eight perma-caths in my chest and a tube in my arm that had to be reopened six times because it stopped working.

I then tried peritoneal dialysis for six months. This type of dialysis is where a tube is put into the lower abdominal area behind the peritoneal wall. I had to have the first tube taken out because I developed a hole in my abdominal wall. I had a second tube put in after the hole healed. I had to have this one taken out because it was not working anymore. I had to go back on hemodialysis. By this time I was about to give up on life itself.

I was so depressed and was thinking about suicide because I could not take the surgeries and the pain anymore. I had four people tested to be a match for a kidney transplant for me. My mom was not a match for me. The doctors said she could do it, but it would be risking both our lives. So we decided to wait a little longer.

April 2003 was when my waiting finally ended. One of my mother's friends was a match for me. I jumped for joy! It was my chance to live again. I felt like a weight had been lifted off my shoulders. I went to all my doctors to tell them I could not wait. I went to the dialysis unit to tell them I was not going to be coming back for a long time.

The day of the surgery was scary. They had me walk into the operating room. I was wide awake so I saw all the tools they were going to use. My nerves began to kick in more than I had ever felt them before. I hopped up onto the operating table and let the nurses take over. Soon I was fast asleep. All I remember is waking up to my mom saying I actually looked like a person, not a ghost.

It took awhile for me to recover, but I was up and walking within three days of surgery. I was sore, but I was feeling so good. The medications they had me on were tremendous, and so were the side effects. I was taking almost forty pills a day. I am not one for taking pills, but I had to get used to it. There were so many patients in the hospital that the nurses were kept very busy. My mom visited everyday, and she took even better care of me than the nurses did.

I spent two very long weeks in the hospital. By the time I was released I was walking great and doing very well. I amazed everyone with my speedy recovery. Even though when I got home I was still on bed rest, at least I felt alive and not married to a dialysis machine.

It has been almost two years now since my kidney transplant. I am doing better than ever. I am down to fourteen pills a day. I am in college studying nursing, and living my life like I have wanted to live it. I feel that the only things that kept me alive and hanging in there through my tough times were my friends and my church. Going through all the surgeries, my depression, and hard times has made me a stronger person. I do get tired now and then, but it is because of my medication.

My goal in life is to be a nurse and a motivational speaker. I want people to benefit through my experiences and hard times. That way they can see that even though life throws you a curve ball you can always catch it and turn it around.

Always remember to tell the ones that matter most in your life that you love them because you never know when that curve ball is going to be thrown. When it is, always know that you can overcome anything that is thrown your way.

Claude Garneau
Eosinophilic Fasciitis
Canada

I am a forty-four-year-old male from Ottawa, Canada. In the late spring or early summer of 2003, my wife noticed some red splotches on my lower legs. These would turn black and blue and would then reappear at a later date. She told me to mention this to my doctor. I did so in passing when I went for my annual check-up. I did not put any emphasis on this, as they did not bother me and I felt fine. My doctor thought they might be allergies, and suggested I try an antihistamine. I did, it did not help, and I forgot about the splotches since they did not bother me.

Later during the summer, we went on a cycling holiday. I could not ride more than twenty kilometers without almost dropping dead from exhaustion. (I can usually easily do over one hundred kilometers per day.) Then I started having joint pain and stiffness, as well as extreme fatigue, and I could not get out of a chair without help. Also, I could not kneel down. I lost over twenty-five pounds in a few weeks. I could not straighten out my hands or make a fist. I also had muscle cramps in my legs.

At that point, I knew there was something seriously wrong. My family doctor sent me to see a rheumatologist after running a battery of other tests to eliminate cancer and other things that might be the source of the problems. The rheumatologist felt it was either scleroderma or eosinophilic fasciitis (EF). They did a deep biopsy in my calf, and I was diagnosed with EF.

The doctor started treating me with a couple of medications. These did a good job of keeping my flexibility problem from getting worse and they even helped bring back a little flexibility, but not much. The biggest change was in my fatigue level, where I felt tremendous improvement. However, the disease has kept spreading. I have it all over my body, including in my throat, on my torso, and on my back. I take a potassium supplement that helps with the cramps. I still get cramps in my legs and back, but much less than before.

I also experience a very painful sensation on the front of my feet, at the ankle level. It feels as if I have been scalded. Having socks touch my feet is very painful. A dermatologist prescribed a cream, which did not help. She then did some research and found that some people with immune system disorders develop a condition similar to mine. She prescribed an anti-seizure medication, which seemed to be working very well. I was getting some genuine relief. At about the same time, my rheumatologist added a new medication to try to stop the spread of the disease. After one dose, two days after my first dose, my neutrophil count, a type of white blood cell that fights infection, dropped to zero. They stopped all medication except for one, while they tried to find out the cause of the neutrophil drop. My neutrophil count has since come back to normal levels, but this latest episode only started a few weeks ago, so I do not know the cause of the problem.

I really hope they find out what is causing this, as I am rapidly regressing to the point I was at last summer. My fatigue is coming back, and the inflexibility is now back to where it was last summer. This is getting a little discouraging.

Lori Schultz
Eosinophilic Fasciitis
Georgia, USA

My daughter, Lindsey, age fifteen, has been a diabetic since she was five years old. Since late last fall 2002, she has complained of fatigue and muscle soreness. I thought this was because she was not getting enough sleep, so I brushed it off.

Early this winter she showed me her arms and legs and they felt very hard. I rushed her to the doctor who was very concerned, but I was told by the head of pediatric endocrinology that this was a condition common in children with uncontrolled diabetes.

As a mother, I felt compelled to get a second opinion. During my appointment with her endocrinologist I mentioned her arms and legs and he said she needs to see a rheumatologist. The first visit to the rheumatologist was extensive. She knew my daughter had some connective tissue disease but was uncertain whether it was scleroderma or scleredema.

The rheumatologist consulted a dermatologist who did a biopsy, which came back inconclusive, so a second one was done. They went further into the fascia and confirmed the diagnosis of eosinophilic fasciitis (EF).

She was initially placed on cimetidine and then methotrexate. She has only been on methotrexate for a month and so far there has been no change. They are holding off the corticosteroid therapy due to the fact she is diabetic.

◆❖◆

Ronald Allinson
Fibrosing Alveolitis
England, UK

I am now sixty-five, and I was diagnosed with fibrosing alveolitis in October 1996. Since then I have spent a lot of time in the hospital, including six weeks in intensive care.

I have also suffered a pneumothorax to the left lung that took over twelve days to re-inflate. I get very breathless just moving about. I also suffer from cervical and lumber spondylosis, osteoarthritis and osteopenia.

I cannot get around without a wheelchair. I drive a specially adapted estate car which has an automatic wheelchair hoist.

My local National Health System Trust has been very supportive as has my hospital physician, who is the most caring person I have ever met.

I am on a high dosage of steroids, along with other medication. I also have oxygen at home and a portable cylinder when I go out. I use a nebulizer four times a day, and a respiratory nurse visits me once a month.

My wife and two daughters and two sons-in-laws have also been very supportive. They are as aware as I am that I am very lucky to still be here. I am a very positive person, to the point where my family calls me a stubborn old guy.

Lenor Fowler
Pulmonary Fibrosis
Connecticut, USA

Up until 1999, I considered myself a very healthy person. All that changed in May 1999 when I was diagnosed with polymyositis and Raynaud's phenomenon. In March of 2001, I was diagnosed with pulmonary fibrosis.

In September 1998 my hands and neck became very stiff. I thought it was due to yard work so, of course, I ignored it. Weeks went by and my condition was not getting any better, so I went to my chiropractor in order to work out these kinks. She told me I should be tested for Lyme disease. Even though I never saw any evidence of a tick bite, this made sense to me since I had been outside doing lots of yard work and Connecticut is an area where there have been many occurrences of the disease. I had my doctor test me for Lyme and he put me on antibiotics that day. The test results were inclusive. By that time I was starting to feel worse. I found it hard to sit down, and walking up stairs was impossible.

In October, I went to see a doctor who specialized in Lyme disease. He began my treatment by ruling out what I did not have. The first disease to be eliminated from the list of possibilities was meningitis. On Christmas Eve 1998, I went in for a spinal tap. It came back negative, which was good news—no meningitis! The next step was to send me to a rheumatologist to rule out any disorders in that field. My story might have been very different had this doctor not missed the polymyositis. He concurred with the diagnosis of my other doctors and sent me on my way.

My liver tests remained elevated, to about three times the norm. Even though all of my tests came back as positive-negative, or inconclusive, the only thing they could come up with was Lyme Disease.

In April 1999, the doctors put me on an intravenous (IV) broad-spectrum antibiotic for nine weeks with the hopes that this treatment would be effective, as all other antibiotics had failed. After the ninth week I still was not any better. I found it hard to breathe and swallow, and walking was almost impossible. I needed help getting to and from the bathroom and the bedroom.

All the while I continued to work. When I traveled I checked into handicapped rooms and asked for wheelchair assistance at airports. I felt so bad and cried alot, which was very unusual for me. My whole body hurt. I felt like I was ninety, but I was only thirty-six. I just kept thinking, "I have to keep going or I will lose everything I worked so hard for."

I continued to search for answers about my condition and on May 21, 1999, I went to see a liver specialist at Yale University School of Medicine. He asked me if I had ever been tested for HIV. My first thought was, "Great, I have AIDS. How am I going to get through this?" My answer was no. He admitted me to the hospital that day for testing. My HIV test came back negative. However, my CPK (blood test for creatine phosphokinase) was 11,200 (normal is 55 to 127). It was at this time that I was diagnosed with polymyositis. I never had Lyme disease. They confirmed the polymyositis with a muscle biopsy on May 24th. I was so happy that they had finally diagnosed the problem. I am going to live! Polymyositis is not life threatening unless there is lung involvement, and I did not have that! I was released from the hospital on May 25th with a prescription of 60mg of prednisone per day. I was on the road to recovery, or so I thought.

I found a new rheumatologist and started treatment for polymyositis. He started me on methotrexate. My CPK levels went up and down over the next two years and I developed Raynaud's phenomenon. My dry cough came back some time in February 2001, but I adjusted to my new life. I could not do everything I had done before I got sick. My mountain biking and rock climbing days were definitely over, but I was grateful I was not in any pain. I moved around more like an old lady than a thirty-seven-year-old, but I was okay with that.

On March 3, 2001, my world came to a halt when my doctors discovered I had developed pulmonary fibrosis while on the methotrexate treatment for polymyositis. My rheumatologist sent me to a pulmonologist and he confirmed the disease. He told me I had to treat my health like my second career. Great, like I did not have enough to deal with already. I did not want my health to be my second career. I just wanted to wake up and feel good and now I knew that that was never going to happen. I went home and looked up pulmonary fibrosis and what I discovered was not good. Everything I found came up with the same prognosis of three to six years, and lung transplants. I felt like I had just been given a prison term with no hope for parole. I went all the way down into depression. The doctors added an antidepressant to my long prescription list, and also switched me from methotrexate to an immunosuppressant that is less toxic on the lungs.

And as if that was not enough, in November 2001, I ended the six year relationship with my boyfriend. So much for that support! Needless to say, December was tough, but I love a good challenge.

In February 2002, the immunosuppressant was not working and I was scared something else was going to go wrong, so I pushed the doctors for something new. They put me on intravenous immunoglobulin (IVIG) therapy. On March 12, 2002, I received my first treatment. I started to feel better and over time my CPKs went down to 267 and my medications were lowered. I lost twenty-five pounds and was feeling great. I had no breathing problems or cough. The lung test remained the same and I felt and looked better than I had in years. I even went off the antidepressant.

On April 13, 2002, I had my first date in over seven years. Chris was unbelievable! A dream come true. Not only was he the most compassionate and thoughtful person I had ever met, he was also great looking and in great shape. On our first date I explained my medical problems to him, and to his credit he was still up for the challenge of a second date. He has been by my side ever since. He is my angel.

In January 2003 I turned forty. Chris and I went on vacation for two weeks. It was a trip I will never forget. It was also the first time I had ever taken two weeks off in a row from work. I felt great and never coughed and I got lots of rest.

When I returned home, I went in for a breathing test. In six months I had lost ten percent more of my lung capacity. I had somewhere between forty-eight and thirty-eight percent lung capacity left, so I was switched to another medication.

It was also time to really make changes in my life. This was a turning point for me, as I was inspired to post a web site. It is called Lenor's Journey because that is exactly what it has been, a journey! I want to share my experience to let others know, as I do, they are not the only ones dealing with this. My goal in life is to live it one day at a time.

◆ ❖ ◆

David G. Burt
Raynaud's
England, UK

I am fifty-one years old and suffer from Raynaud's, bipolar affective disorder, high anxiety and phobias for which I am unable to take medication due to severe side effects. I am slim for my height, which is 5' 10." During the late fall, winter and early spring seasons I experience extreme cold, and aching in my hands, arms and lower legs in an ambient temperature of anything less than 65° Fahrenheit (18° Celsius). This is often made far worse when I am depressed or anxious, which causes my body temperature to drop by a degree or so.

Any sudden upset can leave me shivering with cold and cause my fingers to go white, even when the ambient temperature is reasonably warm. I have noticed that when ambient temperatures are cold at night, I wake up with a temperature of around 95° F (35° C), and I feel more comfortable than would be expected. This sensation leaves as soon as I take warm food or fluid, and then I start to shiver and the pain in my limbs returns.

I have found that the only cure for this is to increase my blood temperature by strenuous exercise or by bathing in water that is not too hot. Bathing can take as long as thirty minutes before I feel comfortably warm, and this comfort can soon go if the ambient temperature is not high enough.

My doctor has recommended in the past that I take a holiday in a warmer country such as Spain or Italy during the coldest part of winter, but this has not always been possible. I suffered the same symptoms as a child, when I was at a private boarding school in England whilst my parents lived in the tropics. I suffered very bad chilblains as well as the other symptoms I still experience throughout the colder months, but my symptoms would disappear as if by magic whenever I landed in South America.

In order to ease my discomfort when the ambient temperature is low, I wrap up as warmly as possible, with as many layers as possible, especially on my limbs. I try to avoid going outside when temperatures are lower than about 40° F (4.5° C), or if there is a severe chill factor in the wind.

I try to remember that I will feel much better come April, but the pain of feeling cold can severely add to my depression.

◆❖◆

Diana Brown
Raynaud's
Canada

I am not sure what happened to me. I did not ask any questions nor was I looking for any answers. I was tired of going to the doctor and being told it was from stress. When I finally did go for help, I had let things go too far and all I wanted was to get back to normal. I did everything I was told, but when I figured the doctor had given up on me because he could not explain things, I took matters into my own hands. I stopped the medication because I felt it was hurting me more than it was helping me. I was in bad shape, but I got to the point where it was up to me to push myself back to a more normal life.

Five of my finger tips turned black and I lost control of my hands. My legs and feet swelled like balloons. My arms and shoulders hurt. I could lift my arms above my head, but someone else had to bring them back down for me. I lost strength in my hands and arms. I walked like I was ninety years old. There was not a part of my body that did not hurt.

The specialist that I was sent to was amazed with my fingers and I don't think he had ever seen this before. He got a bunch of doctors together so they could all examine my hands to see if they knew what was wrong with me. One of the doctors had been treating a patient who had the same thing for the last six months, but still they did not know what they were dealing with. This specialist dealt only with my fingers, and some of the medication he put me on caused my legs to swell even more. I complained about the swelling, but he said he was more worried I would lose the fingers; so he took care of the fingers first.

He diagnosed me with acrocyanosis, not Raynaud's, because of the length of time the fingers stayed black. They were black for six to seven weeks. I was tested for lupus, rheumatoid arthritis and fibromyalgia. I had a lot of the symptoms of fibromyalgia, but he could not positively diagnose it as that. So I was never actually told much, but as my hands got better I was sent to another doctor for the legs and feet. She did all her tests and could not come up with any diagnosis either, so I was sent back to the family doctor.

I fought for two years with the swollen legs and feet until my doctor had a student in with him who thought of trying something new. I was on fluid pills but there is another medication that is taken half an hour before the fluid pill and it is the first thing that has actually helped.

My hands have never turned black again. Now they turn ghostly white, feel numb, and burn. Then they change to dark red before they return to normal. I have the same color changes with my feet. I think this is Raynaud's, but I am waiting to see the specialist.

My younger sister was having trouble with one fingertip that is staying black so I went the specialist with her, which is the same specialist that I am waiting to see. I am normally a very shy, quiet person but this was a chance to learn things, so I asked what her diagnosis was.

When I was told it was Raynaud's, I made a point of describing the difference between acrocyanosis and Raynaud's. I might have stepped over the line, but I knew the difference. When the doctor returned, he made a point of not saying what it was because the intern had told him what I said. He just said that the tests had not all come back yet. My sister's finger will likely be back to normal when we go back on Tuesday, so I want to see if they will continue testing to find the cause of her symptoms, since she has had this happen two other times. However, this is the first time she was sent to the specialist and the longest her finger has remained black.

Right now my body is sore all over. When I first noticed a difference in my hands, arms and shoulders, I was put on a medication. Within three weeks my whole body was sore, so I returned to the doctor and was put on another medicine. It took me almost three years to get the acrocyanosis diagnosis since I was never told what they thought I had. Unless you ask, they certainly do not volunteer any information.

Hopefully I will be seen by the specialist soon and get some answers to my problems. Maybe they will review my records and find something.

My problems do not even come close to what others are going through. I have been reading the stories and I can see how so many people are much worse off than I am. I hope everyone receives all the help they need. My prayers are with you all.

❖❖❖

Helen Paschali
Raynaud's
Cyprus

I first had Raynaud's, which is the changing color of hands accompanied with numb and tingly feelings, seven years ago. A year later I had all the same symptoms, but this time also with swelling and about three big ulcers on each finger.

I went to several doctors who told me I had chilblains and I was not to worry. But as the years went on the pain was getting worse and worse. I still had all the above symptoms, but now even worse pain.

Every time winter comes, I dread it, as I know what I am going to go through. I saw a specialist in the United Kingdom, who diagnosed me with Raynaud's. I knew I had Raynaud's and kept telling the doctors over here, but they told me I was crazy! I knew that a chilblain could not possibly cause the kind of pain that I had.

This winter, however, was different. I had all the usual symptoms, but I could not make a fist and could not do simple things like brush my teeth or button up my shirt! I have a family to look after and try not to let it stop me from caring for them, but I cannot express how painful this is.

If by accident I should bang my hand, I feel like I will pass out from the pain. Also this year I have pain in my elbows and knees. I do not want to see a doctor again just to hear him tell me that I have chilblains and that they will pass on their own!

Do I have scleroderma? Does it make a difference if one catches it early?

John G.
Raynaud's
New Jersey, USA

I am a heavy equipment mechanic by trade and come in contact with cold steel on a daily basis. I thought the cold steel was the problem, but it is not. If I walk out to the mailbox across the front lawn for just a few seconds, my hands turn a greenish white color and become numb.

The cold only affects my hands and feet. Even in the slightest cold weather I lose the ability to use my hands, and it has made it very difficult to function.

I am forty-five and this has been getting worse as the years go by. My doctor tells me to keep warm, but I wonder if something else is wrong that he is not telling me.

I have learned to live with this and thought I was the only person with this problem. Even with gloves on I cannot stay out in the cold for long. I am in very good shape otherwise. I exercise daily, do not smoke and have a good diet.

Other than keeping warm as the doctor told me to do, which is impossible at my job, I do not know what else to do. I have to work outside when we have snowstorms, and when there are equipment breakdowns. My boss thinks I am making excuses. It is hard to convince people who do not have Raynaud's that it is real and that it has an effect on people.

Carlo Hernandez
Scleroderma or Multiple Sclerosis
Venezuela

This story was translated from Italian to English by Kevin Howell. He is a Clinical Scientist for Professor Carol Black at the Royal Free Hospital in London. The Italian version of this story is in Chapter 10.

In 1997 I caught a bad cold, and after a week I was walking along and lost my balance. I was talking as if I was drunk, with pains in the legs, arms and head every day. After four weeks they referred me to a neurologist, who checked me over and told me I had the symptoms of multiple sclerosis (MS).

I took 1 gm solumedrol for 5 days, and recovered by 60%. On the MRI I had no plaques on the brain or the medulla. I had neuropathy at the left eye, and the EMG showed a small abnormality at the left eye and the left ear. I used to be a pilot for an airline here in Venezuela. I am also Italian through my mother.

I lost my pilot's licence because of this episode. Nowadays my doctor is a bit confused because she tells me that I have symptoms that are not associated with multiple sclerosis—for example I have always had pain for almost seven years—and she tells me that for this condition I ought to have plaques on the brain.

I would like to know if it could be cerebellar thoracic outlet syndrome or Raynaud's which is associated with the sclerosis.

◆ ❖ ◆

Patty Sandoval Sralla
Sjögren's Syndrome
Michigan, USA

It all started with a rusty nail, at least that is my theory.

I was eight years old, unafraid, full of energy and curiosity. My mother told me to wear sandals whenever I played outside. Like most children, I disobeyed now and then. That bright summer day was one of those times when I ventured outside without shoes. I was running through a field of long grass playing with some friends, unaware of the debris in my path. I stepped on a board with an old rusty nail sticking out of it. The nail went in and out of my foot. I ran to the house and ran water from a water hose over the wound as blood gushed out. Afraid of getting in trouble, I found a rag in the garage and wrapped my foot until the bleeding stopped. I did not tell my mother.

A couple of days later, I woke up with my knee the size of a grapefruit. It was full of liquid and I could not straighten it out without extreme pain. My mother rushed me to the doctor's office. They drained the fluid with a big syringe. My mother almost passed out. I was admitted to the hospital with a massive infection. I was given three shots three times a day of antibiotics. I will never forget how I dreaded those injections. I stayed there for a week or so and was sent home on crutches, with more antibiotics. I recovered quickly and soon returned to my normal schedule.

A few months later I developed fluid-filled bumps on my wrists. The doctor removed the fluid by syringe once or twice a month. I had to take aspirin for inflammation until it cleared up.

After that I started to get little white patches of dry skin on my left upper arm. I showed them to my mother. She applied creams including aloe vera, but it did not work. The patches started to connect and harden. We went to our family doctor who thought it was a fungus. We applied anti-fungal medication. It did not help. The patches spread down the inside of my arm toward my hand. My family doctor suspected an arthritis-related illness. He said I should take aspirin.

My parents were not content with that answer so they took me to the Kelsey-Sebold Clinic in Houston. There, I underwent lots of tests including a barium X ray and a biopsy of my arm. They diagnosed me with localized scleroderma and said there was no treatment as the disease had to run its course. They said I should take massive doses of aspirin and Vitamin E.

Meanwhile, the hardening spread to my left thumb and started to spread up toward my neck as well. I exercised with a rubber ball to keep my thumb from atrophying. It did not work. My left thumb was left small and disabled. The creeping hardening of the skin continued its crawl up my shoulder and then it stopped. The white patches now had an odd brownish pigment and the muscle underneath was clearly disfigured. I was twelve years old. For the next twenty five years, I lived my life with this scar from my shoulder to my hand. Though it was hard growing up with this en coupe de sabre, as this form of scleroderma is called, I knew I was lucky. I was healthy otherwise and did all the things young women do. I was active in school, had boyfriends, went to college, got married, had two children, and enjoyed a successful career as a journalist.

Then around the age of thirty-six, I started noticing that I was having shortness of breath when I exercised. Though I was always about fifteen to twenty pounds overweight, I could always exercise and get down to my 'fighting' weight of one hundred and twenty pounds. But this was different; I would exercise and feel worse afterwards. I could not get through long exercise tapes without feeling breathless and extra tired. I chalked it up to getting older.

Each year during my checkup I would mention it to the doctor. He would listen to my lungs and heart and say it might be stress from work. I started trying to reduce my stress but it didn't seem to help. I started feeling more and more fatigued. So when I went in for my yearly checkup on my thirty-seventh birthday, I again told my doctor about the shortness of breath and fatigue. He listened to my heart and this time he heard something. He brought in an EKG machine and saw the telltale signs of the right side of my heart working extra hard.

That is when I first heard the words pulmonary hypertension (PH). He said that people with scleroderma can get PH, which is a rare cardiovascular disorder caused by high blood pressure in the pulmonary arteries. "One out of a million," he said. But people with my type of scleroderma, linear scleroderma, are not supposed to get PH. So he sent me to a lung specialist, a rheumatologist and a cardiologist.

After several more tests, the new lung doctor said my lungs were the healthiest he had seen in a long time. "No PH," he declared.

The rheumatologist tested my blood for scleroderma, lupus, and other autoimmune antibodies. I tested negative for scleroderma or lupus, but came up positive for Sjögren's, an autoimmune disease that affects the glands in the eyes and mouth. This made sense, because I had been having trouble with eye dryness. I went to see an eye doctor who told me to use a different type of eye drop that can be purchased over the counter. The drops helped, but my tongue began to develop cracks and hurt when I ate certain foods. This is also a symptom of Sjögren's.

The rheumatologist concluded that I did not have any signs of systemic scleroderma. Although I had struggled with heartburn most of my life, tests showed no signs of scleroderma in my esophagus.

During that time, I also saw Dr. Maureen Mayes, who is an internationally known expert on scleroderma. She was still in Detroit at the time and concluded that I did not have active scleroderma.

However, the cardiologist said I had PH and that the prognosis was not good. I had mean pulmonary pressures of about 78, which indicates moderate to severe pulmonary hypertension, and my pulse oxygen rate reduced to 85 when I stood up.

I decided to get a second opinion with a local expert in PH, Dr. Mel Rubenfire, a cardiologist who runs the Pulmonary Hypertension Clinic at the University of Michigan (U-M). I met Dr. Rubenfire a few months later. He confirmed the diagnosis of PH but gave me hope. He also didn't think that it was related to the scleroderma but he could not rule it out. Either I had a rare case of childhood linear scleroderma developing internal involvement years later or I was struck by lightning twice. Regardless, it was a serious condition and we had to do something about it soon.

I had a right heart catherization to get an exact measurement and to see if I responded to another type of medication. I did not respond to the oral medication so they started me on the strongest blood vessel dilator, which is administered by IV twenty-four hours a day. I was set up with a Hickman catheter in my chest, shown how to mix my medicine daily, how to keep from getting infections, and how to deal with side effects of the medication.

At first, it was scary, but the medicine really helped with my quality of life. I was already at the point where I could not walk up stairs without being winded. I was sleeping all weekend and I couldn't think very straight. Once the medication started, it was like a new day for me. I had not felt that good in such a long time that it made the side effects easy to handle. I had nausea, migraine headaches, diarrhea, jaw pain, leg pain, and acid reflux. I was still working full-time and juggling the boys with the help of my husband.

Though the treatment helped me and had the potential to restore some of the damage in the blood vessels, I was not getting better. A second heart catherization a year later revealed that the pressure in my pulmonary arteries was getting worse. They started talking to me about heart and lung transplants. I was devastated.

The transplant team at the University of Michigan wanted assurances that I didn't have scleroderma, so I had to return to the rheumatologist for more blood work. When I retested more than a year later, the results were reversed; I tested positive for scleroderma antibodies and negative for Sjögren's. The rheumatologist and Dr. Mayes both thought that the blood test had been incorrectly processed.

At this point, I was pretty desperate. I did not want to have a transplant. So I called up Dr. Rubenfire and we talked about other options. He said we could push the IV medication as much as I could handle and see what happens. I agreed. I also decided to pull out all the stops and try just about every alternative therapy I had heard about, working with a doctor and a certified practitioner.

In May 2001, I returned to the University of Michigan for another right heart catherization. My pressures had reduced to a mean of 55! I was so excited. The doctor at U-M said that the increased IV medication might have had something to do with it. Also, they discovered something new during this cath: I had a large atrial septal defect; which is a hole in my heart. The doctor is not sure whether the hole caused the PH or if it opened up to relieve the pressure. Either way, it explained why my oxygen levels dropped so significantly when I walked. It was also a better explanation than scleroderma, which did not make sense to anyone. With the reduced pressures I became a good candidate for a new oral drug for PH which is an endothelial antagonist that prevents inflammation in the blood vessels. I started it in June 2001 but it made me feel so bad at first that I stopped taking it.

I continued with a myriad of alternative therapies throughout the summer. Overall, I felt about the same, though I was able to do yoga and walk on my treadmill.

In September 2002, I saw my U-M doctor again and my six minute walk was the best I had ever done. I did not need oxygen and I walked farther.

The echocardiogram estimated my pressures at about the same, mid-50s. I was having a lot of acid reflux as a result of the increased IV medication as well. So the doctor suggested I give the new medication another try. I started taking it at a lower dose. I felt the same side effects, but they subsided after a few days. We increased the dose and I have been on it for about five months now. In this time, I have been able to reduce my IV medication to where I was when I started.

I have quit my job and reduced my stress one hundred percent. I am doting on my children and my husband. I am calling my parents more often and talking to my sisters and brother at least once a week. I am also seeking out long lost friends.

There is no more putting off for tomorrow in my world. I am writing a screenplay, which is something I have always wanted to do. I am working with some nonprofit organizations to help the poor.

I have learned that time is indeed fleeting and that we all have only limited time to learn and do well. Then it is time to move on and go back to God. No matter what the outcome, I have learned to take control and I am not afraid anymore. That is a lot to learn in three years, all before my fortieth birthday. And that is the beauty of it.

D.M.
Undiagnosed
Kosovo, Yugoslavia

I am a twenty-five and a student of medicine at St. Vincent's. Not long ago my mother was sick and I took her to an internal disease doctor.

She had hypertension, arthritis, and bronchitis. He noticed that the skin on the upper part of her arms is thick. He assumed it was scleroderma. He recommended another doctor here in Kosovo who is a specialist in that area. I went with my mother to see that doctor and he stated that she had scleroderma, without any analyses or further consultation.

My mother has always had thick skin, so I asked him, "Why do you think this is scleroderma?" He was not very friendly and he said, as usually the doctors in Kosovo do, "This is it." He said she had diffuse progressive systemic sclerosis, and he recommended several medications.

I fully disagreed with him, because the color of my mother's skin has not changed. She is feeling okay and she does not feel any pain. She does not have any deformation in the face or body in general. She can swallow without any problem. I also disagreed with him because he made that conclusion without taking blood tests.

He then recommended that she take the following blood tests: immunoglobulines, C3 and C4, and sedimentation. He also ordered a spirometry of the esophagus (esophageal manometry).

I did my best to have these tests done for my mother even though these tests are very expensive here in Kosovo. The analyses were all in the range of normal. When we saw the doctor the next time, we showed him the analyses and he said that they were all right, but he never changed the diagnosis.

I went with my mother to another doctor some one thousand miles away and this doctor said, "No. I fully disagree with the other one because this is not scleroderma." He is an old experienced doctor and he said that he can recognize the patients with scleroderma when he sees them entering his clinic.

I also consulted some other doctors and none of them agreed with that diagnosis. Please help me and tell me what I should do. I will do my best to help my mother. She is the only person I have in this world.

❖❖❖

Fionna Paton
Undiagnosed
Australia

My problems began in 1999 (when I was thirty-six), after a particularly stressful year. I had joint pain in my fingers so I had a blood test. My anti-nuclear antibody (ANA) test was positive a 1:160, and they thought I had lupus. I was retested a few weeks later and the results were normal.

A few months after that I started having numbness in my arms and legs and I became extremely cold intolerant. One day I noticed that it felt like blood was rushing in and out of my hands. Eventually it got so bad that I had it checked out and I was diagnosed with Raynaud's.

About a year later my hands started to change. The skin thickened on my right index finger and my other fingers became like putty. If I pinch the skin between my fingers and then let it go, the skin stays there for quite some time without springing back into shape.

My fingers also are much fatter than they were. My rings no longer fit properly. I usually wake up with very swollen fingers and 'pins and needles' so bad I cannot move my arms. My arms get sore even when I just blow dry my hair or raise them above my head. My hands go numb doing simple things like putting on makeup or using a knife and fork.

A few months ago I started getting heartburn. It is quite painful, and at first I thought I must be having a heart attack. I also have trouble brushing my teeth without vomiting because of the reflux.

I am very fatigued, but all my tests done come back okay. My general practitioner believes I have scleroderma but she does not know which type. I haven't been to rheumatologist for a while. Unless there is a symptom they can see, or certain antibodies, they think there is nothing wrong. The only constant has been my last four or five ANA tests that have all been positive in a nuclear pattern with a titer of 1:160.

I know there is something very wrong with me, but unless the blood tests precisely reveal it, it will be a long, long road to a diagnosis. I am very frustrated by all of this and feel that I should be getting treatment now, before it gets worse.

◆❖◆

Lee
Undiagnosed
Florida, USA

Five months ago my fingers were suddenly started tingling and became a bit swollen. I didn't think much of it at first, but it persisted for two months so I went to my doctor. He didn't know what it was and referredme to a neurologist.

The neurologist also didn't know what it was. With no help from my primary doctor, I talked it over with a few people and finally decided to see a rheumatologist.

The rheumatologist did blood tests, which came back normal except for a positive antinuclear antibody (ANA) result of 1:640. I was given a short of cortisone and sent h ome with anti-inflammatory medications. None of it helped.

I did some homework before I saw the rheumatologist again, and I asked about plaquenil. It has given me a lot of relief from my symptoms, but my fingers are still very swollen, hard, painful and difficult to work with.

I saw some other specialists who think I may have scleroderma, but they cannot swear to it. My systemic scleroderma blood test came back negative. Now I am waiting for my limited scleroderma test to see if that is positive or negative.

CHAPTER 8

Overlap, UCTD and
MCTD Stories

*If we try to feel positive about our life
and the cards we are dealt, then we can
manage our disease most effectively.*

—Silezia Pretorius

Charmaine E. Collings
Michigan, USA

My first symptom began as a little spot that looked like a purple bruise, the size of a quarter on the front top of my left leg.

After it had been there for a month, I asked my doctor if he thought this bruise, which would not go away, was anything to be concerned about. The first thing he said was, "Well, I do not think it is a bruise." This was a pretty big surprise to me. In response to further questions from me he indicated that he did not know what it was, and that maybe I should see a dermatologist.

I was being treated at the time for anal fissures, as well as what seemed, at the time, to be a yeast infection. Later, those two problems together would be diagnosed as lichen sclerosus, something I have often wondered if it had anything to do with the diagnosis of scleroderma.

Soon multiple spots developed across my abdomen, with a few stray ones on my forearms and more on the left leg. Today, nearly two years after the first spot showed up, the spots continue to spread. The older ones—some very large, hard ones that are the shape of a cucumber, on both of my hips—have become leathery, and the centers have turned ivory in color. In general, they do not bother me, but the largest one (which is about eight inches in length, and about three inches wide, on my hip) has become tender underneath.

Sometimes the skin's outermost layer feels flaky and dry, causing me to hope that they will just disappear by peeling off! That is not happening, but they are not very attractive, and I do dream about having clear skin again someday. I have not read enough about other people's experiences to know if that is even a possibility, but a girl can hope!

I have read in different places that this condition can appear to go into remission, anywhere from three to...drum roll...twenty-five years later. Three years sounds good, but twenty-five years makes me feel like this will be with me until I die, since I am fifty-two years old. I have read that even if the spots stop spreading, the damage done to the skin is permanent. This was not good news, so I have had to adjust my thinking and decide not to let any of it bother me. Sometimes it is difficult to ignore it.

I wear long sleeves, and I try to tan to camouflage the spots, but in general, I try not to think about them. Still, they are there, they are noticeable, and they continue to spread. I am heavy, and I used to not want people to see my bare abdomen since I felt self-conscious because of its largeness. Now, I run my hands over my middle as I lay in bed at night, remembering what the smooth unblemished skin looked like, and I wish I could have it back.

My clothing irritates my hips where it rests directly on the lumpy skin, but other than that I have not had terrible problems. I have been tested (lungs, heart, and esophagus) to see if it was scleroderma (originally diagnosed by the dermatologist as morphea). The rheumatologist who ordered those tests and did a physical exam lists three versions of scleroderma that seem to be part of my overall condition: morphea, linear and diffuse. Although the testing on internal organs indicates that I have no damage to them, my doctor, a University of Michigan hospital doctor, has told me he cannot guarantee that those things will not happen in the future. For now I am thankful that I have no more severe damage internally and that it is only skin involvement.

I struggle with trying to discover why I got this. I have read things that indicate different causes, and have a list of things that I can relate to. I had a hip to hip "tummy tuck" surgery, with a repair of an underlying abdominal muscle in 1983. I took the diet drug combo, fen-phen, for far longer than the recommended six weeks. In fact, I took it for one year and this seems like a likely candidate, since there are people who have had damaged heart and lungs and the drugs were consequently removed from the market! I have also looked for environmental causes.

This seems weird to me that I have something which might be a reaction to some toxin, since I never even use spray cans because of my belief that they cause health problems, and I have also tried to avoid pesticides, antibiotics, and other pollutants.

I live in a trailer and I have PVC pipes, and I wonder and worry that this may have caused the problem. In fact, I worry about it so much, that I was trying to drink bottled water exclusively, but I have given that up. I even let my water from my pipes sit out to let the chlorine dissipate before I drink it. I still do this, but what is the point if I do not have to do it all the time?

I had incredible stress in my life several years before advent of the symptoms. It started with a fall at work, resulting in subsequent shoulder surgery for a torn rotator cuff, and then back problems (herniated discs) with such pain that I received multiple injections into the back (facet injections). These injections were a combination of a steroid and painkiller, and I also had an epidural injection. I had these treatments for a year. Then after that happened, I was in an auto accident in 1998 and had wrist surgery, open reduction with hardware, and surgery a year later to remove the hardware. My mother lived with me for a period from 1996, just before the shoulder surgery, to 1997, and then in March of 1998, while I was recovering from the injuries from the auto accident, my mother passed away. In 1996, I visited both my mother and my son, who was exhibiting signs of the same severe mental illness my mother had, in the psychiatric wards of a local hospital.

Ultimately, my son's illness progressed, and he committed suicide. This happened right after I found out that the post office would not reassign me (because of some loss of wrist mobility I asked to be reassigned to a job not requiring delivery duties and driving), but were going to force me to retire on a disability (my only disability at the time was not being able to bend my left wrist backwards). I had lost my son, which was an incredible tragedy, and incredibly painful, but now I also had no job, no income, and struggled to get public assistance as I looked for other work.

I do receive a small retirement pension, but it is insufficient to live on, and I do have a so-called "temporary" job with Manpower, and have been on the same assignment for nearly three years. In some ways I feel lucky to have any work at all, but in others, the instability of my circumstances (job could end any day), and not being too attractive to a prospective employer with the health issues (sometimes I think it is my age, or my weight, but I also think they must know about the scleroderma, although I try to hide with long sleeves, as it does not affect my abilities to type, file, etc. right now, although my hands are not able to completely close, I can type and file, keyboards are still within my range of motion), gets me down.

I worry about my hands eventually being totally immobile. I cannot make a fist, nor totally open the right hand, which makes me prone to drop things, and makes it difficult to hold a blow dryer, or even to take hold of things being handed to me at a drive-up window (banking, fast food, dry cleaning).

I would be very happy to hear from someone with similar symptoms and related issues. Thank you for allowing me to share some information about my experience with this very baffling condition.

❖❖❖

Daniel B. K.
Virginia, USA

Two months after I was born the doctors noticed that my growth rate was very slow. Unknown to my mother the doctors made a note in my medical chart that my mom was not feeding me. Of course, this was not true.

As time went on it became apparent that my growth rate was not normal. My body was very stiff and rigid so my mother took me back to the doctor and my first biopsy was performed. At this time I was diagnosed with scleroderma and my parents were told that this was a terminal disease.

At age six I was referred to the National Institute of Health in Washington D.C. to see if I was a candidate for growth hormone treatment. It was decided that I was not. Also the doctors were not sure if my diagnosis was correct. I was developing severe contractures in my legs and also my left foot was deformed. The next course of treatment was to place my left leg in a cast. Every night my mother was to increase the size of the wedge behind my knee. It was so painful that the whole idea was discontinued. At this point the doctors could not decide what my diagnosis was.

We went to Bethesda Naval Hospital where the doctors gave me a 'trash can diagnosis', that meant I had a connective tissue disease, however they could not identify which one. This also meant they could treat the symptoms but not the illness.

My next course of treatment began with several surgeries; the first on my left foot to lengthen my heel cord. The second was on my left knee to release my ham strings under my knee. After that I had a total reconstruction on my left foot to improve my walking. This basically was the only surgery that improved my mobility. I continue to have severe contractures in my joints and my mobility is limited. Another surgery was performed on my left knee to limit my contractures in my left leg. It was also mentioned that hip surgery may be needed in the future.

Most doctors I see are interested in the condition when they see me; however, they do not choose to monitor my condition. One doctor dismissed me as a patient because she felt there was nothing she could do to help me. I do, however, have a doctor now that takes an interest in me as a patient. He monitors my lung capacity that at the moment is at fifty-seven percent. I am also at risk for pulmonary fibrosis and need to be checked periodically.

My current health insurance is Medicare and Medicaid. I receive SSDI (Social Security Disability Income). None of my medications are currently being covered. Medicare will not pay for my lung functioning tests, and Medicaid will only pay for my medications when I meet a very large spend down every six months.

I have had several infections in my left foot. I also need regular foot care that is not covered under my Medicare or Medicaid plan. I try to manage my condition as best I can even though my mobility is limited. I do get out and sometimes travel as I am able to drive, but I am uncertain as to what my general health will be in the future.

The one thing I have found about this particular illness is that its progress can not be predetermined.

I manage my life the best I can. And try to enjoy each day. It is important to have a positive outlook on life and remember that we are not alone with this disease.

Donna H.
Pennsylvania, USA

I am a forty-nine, married, and have one son, who will soon be seventeen.

I was diagnosed with Raynaud's in 2001. I was just recently diagnosed with CREST scleroderma in January of 2003. I also have autoimmune hepatitis (AIH), which was confirmed in January 2001, and I have fibromyalgia.

I am very selective who I tell about my diseases, I guess because many people have never heard of some of them and right away when someone looks at you, you just know in the back of your mind, they are thinking, "Is she contagious?" Since most of my problems are autoimmune related, some people will jump to the conclusion that I have AIDS, which is far from the truth.

When I do tell someone about my AIH, right away they think I have regular hepatitis, which can be contagious, but not just by casual contact. AIH is when the body's own immune system attacks the liver. There is no cure, but it is treatable. Some of the symptoms of AIH are the same as symptoms of CREST scleroderma.

I also have other health problems besides the ones listed above, such as degenerative disc disease, osteoarthritis, anxiety/depression/panic disorder, irritable bowel syndrome (IBS), to mention a few. I do seek help with all my diseases, but sometimes it just gets so overwhelming. It feels like I am always at a doctor's office.

I think the thing that I find the hardest about CREST is the itching that I am still getting and all the fatigue because it is dealing with your immune system. I get joint and muscle pain, too. The Raynaud's, which goes along with the CREST, is no walk in the park, either. Winter is bad for me because of the cold, but summer can be too, because of air conditioning. I have found that over the last two years, it is very hard for me to take the heat; I get physically sick and agitated from it.

I am currently seeking the help of a dermatologist for my itching. I just started taking light treatments a few weeks ago. I am to take them at least three times weekly. I just had a dermatologist appointment last week, and told her that I did not think they were helping at all, but she asked me to give them another chance and keep coming for three more weeks until my next appointment.

The past few days, I think I itch a little less, but now my skin is getting drier than usual. I cannot take any pills for the itching with the exception of one, because of my liver problems. Medications can really do a number on the liver if you are not careful and checked all the time.

The CREST affects my right hand more than the left. It constantly looks swollen and it is getting harder and harder for me to even write a check out. I am also getting more pain in my hands and wrists.

I find it very difficult to even keep up with my housework anymore. My husband tries to help out, but he works very long hours. If I am having a good day and do more than I know I should, I suffer for the next few days, sometimes weeks, especially with the fatigue.

My skin starts itching all over, then these little bumps appear, and they still itch to no end. I even scratch until I bleed in my sleep. My husband says I look like a child with the chicken pox. There was a point where they thought I might even have systemic lupus erythematosus (SLE), but my rheumatologist told me it can take a long time to get a correct diagnosis on that. My skin feels tight at times, and I think it is because I am not that advanced yet with the disease. I have red dots on my hands, face and mostly my nose.

I cannot even do dishes without wearing gloves. I have to wear gloves for anything that I might use around the house, like furniture polish or window cleaner, or my fingertips will get worse. So far I have not had any ulcers on my fingertips, but they do get cracked and sore. I find that using a good moisturizer like Eucerin up to three times daily is the best thing for me, more for my hands due to washing them so often. I do not use antibacterial soap anymore. I use Dove soap. I think it works just as well as Aveeno bath and body wash.

I just wish there was something that could be given for the fatigue caused by these autoimmune diseases. The joint pain can get pretty bad too, but if really needed, at least you can take a pain pill for that. And I am still trying to find answers that could help stop the itching. It drives me crazy.

That is about it for now. I will keep you updated on my progress with the light treatments.

Update – September 2003

Since my original story back in May, a lot of things have changed for me. At that time, I was in the process of going for 'light treatments' for my skin, due to all the itching. I gave it additional time like my dermatologist had asked, and it did not help. I had my dermatologist completely stumped. She said that this is not from my scleroderma. She said that I would have patches from morphea, and I tried to tell her that, "I do not have morphea. I have systemic scleroderma with CREST."

Needless to say, she had never heard of that. She even took biopsies that showed nothing. She even went as far as sending me to Hershey Medical Center in Pennsylvania, which is a two and a half hour drive for me.

I was assured by a dermatologist in my area that he would do different testing for my skin, but he did nothing except look at my skin. He kept asking me if I had thyroid problems and if it was checked lately. I told them my thyroid had been checked and the test results are basically normal, sometimes they are off a little, but still within normal ranges.

The doctor at Hershey Medical prescribed two different creams for me, one being a steroid cream, and both are used for psoriasis. I do not have psoriasis, but I must admit, the creams have helped to the point where the itching is bearable.

There was a time, when one Sunday, I was sitting with my husband, Don, and I thought I was going to loose it mentally, the itching just would not stop. I itched all over from top to bottom. Before the trip to Hershey Medical, I spent so much money on different prescriptions and over the counter creams; I could have started my own pharmacy. Before going to Hershey Medical, I saw my rheumatologist, Dr. Miller, for my itching. He agreed it is part of the scleroderma. He also said that there is not much he can do for it but to try to work with the dermatologist to see if he can help me at all. He said the itching could go on for the first couple of years. He also did another pulmonary function test (PFT) and kidney tests. My PFT came back with a slight decline from the last time, but my doctor was not overly concerned yet. My kidney function tests were basically within normal range.

I am at kind of at a loss with the scleroderma, because certain drugs they prescribe for it would be too hard on my liver, and I already have autoimmune hepatitis. Dr. Miller did tell me that when the time comes, he will have to use more aggressive therapy, which I took to mean some type of IV treatment that will bypass the liver more easily. I already take an immune system suppressant drug for my AIH, which we are hoping will also help with the scleroderma.

In the past few months, I have been feeling more fatigued, have had more joint pain, and my hands have been really bothering me to the point that it is difficult to use them like I once did. I have also noticed that occasionally my swallowing is affected. The pain and discomfort I am currently experiencing is really getting to me. I can remember what I could do a year ago, and now it even hurts to clean a mirror or window with my hands. I do wear gloves when my hands touch anything besides regular soap and water, such as chemicals or anything like that.

We did not have a bad summer as far as heat, but when I was outside, the slightest bit would set off my itching, and actually make me feel nauseous and generally miserable. Then I had to be careful inside because of air conditioning affecting my Raynaud's.

My hands are more swollen now, and I also have more skin tightening, especially in the area of the wrist to elbow.

Without a support group, this disease makes you feel totally last, as the doctors do not know everything that can happen to you. My primary care physician asked me if I had asked my rheumatologist for a prognosis. I said, "No, I forgot, but I really do not think it would do any good as everyone is different, and this disease is such a mystery at times."

The doctors seem reluctant to tell you much ahead of time about what might happen and what might not. I think it is due to the fact that they do not even know.

I also have been losing my appetite a lot in the past months. It often takes all I have to get food into me. I usually manage to eat a decent dinner, but prior to dinner, I have no desire to eat. This is completely opposite of how my appetite used to be. I was just told yesterday that I look like I have lost weight. My answer was, "I really do not know how much because I have not been to a doctor to get weighed since July." But within two weeks I will be getting weighed and then I will know. I always wanted to lose weight because I am overweight, but not this way.

I just wish there was something they could do for the fatigue and the pain without using the pain killers that knock me out.

◆✣◆

Jacqueline Smith
California, USA

Ten years ago I moved from British Columbia, Canada to the California desert. For as long as I can remember I have had terribly dry skin and a very hoarse voice with dry mouth. It was tough getting through the music scales with my voice coach. I wanted to pursue a singing career for as long as I can remember, but it is very tough to sing when you have very little moisture in your mouth. My coach said I had a great voice, but it was very hoarse sounding. I even went to Nashville a few times, recorded some songs, but was always held back by this dryness in my throat.

Three years ago, I got this strange rash on my feet. I went to a dermatologist and he took a biopsy and discovered I had morphea, but the other tests were negative. Two years ago I started feeling awful with chest and body pain. I went to see a rheumatologist. He took one look at me and said, "You have lupus. I am sure of that."

He did more blood work and discovered I had overlap syndrome, with systemic lupus erythematosus (SLE), CREST scleroderma, osteoarthritis, Raynaud's, irritable bowel syndrome (IBS), Sjögren's; and I already had hypothyroidism.

The chest pain was getting worse so the rheumatologist suggested I see a cardiologist. He put me through all sorts of tests and said I had minimal heart disease but this was not causing the chest pain. I went to a few different gastroenterologists and had more tests that came back negative. I have pain some days, yet other days I feel fine.

Lately my throat, esophagus, stomach and sternum area have been very painful. I am also having pain in my right ear and temporomandibular joint (TMJ). It has been difficult to open my mouth at times. I have had two endoscopes in the past two years, that came back negative.

I went back to see my rheumatologist, and he said he was sure the scleroderma was in my gastrointestinal tract. I asked him why it was not showing up on the scope and he said, "You have to catch scleroderma at the right time." So who knows?

Next week I am scheduled to see another gastroenterologist. We will see what happens. I get very frustrated with all this. I think everyone thinks I am imagining all of it. I just want to find out what is going on and get on with life. It is very hard to plan anything when I never know how I am going to feel from one day to the next.

Update – May 2003

I went to see another gastroenterologist last Friday, and he performed another endoscope. He discovered scleroderma in my esophagus, as well as an hiatal hernia. This baffles me, as the hiatal hernia did not show up on the other two endoscopes that I had done in the past two years. I realize it is difficult to detect scleroderma in the esophagus, but not a hiatal hernia.

Update – August 2003

I forgot to tell you my age. I do not know if that is important or not, but I am forty-nine and feel ninety-nine! At least now I know why I am having this chest pain.

I have had a laparoscopy and discovered I have severe endometriosis and scleroderma covering the inner lining of my abdomen. I will have to have a complete hysterectomy. When they put me under for the laparoscopy, they had a tough time getting the tube down my throat. My rheumatologist says it is the scleroderma that makes this tough. He says they cannot do much once the skin thickening starts.

Update – November 2003

I saw my rheumatologist yesterday. At first he had told me I had overlap syndrome, but now he says I have just CREST scleroderma. He gave me a shotfor pain and asked me if I would sign up for the consent form for research.

It seems to make it easier when you fall into one illness category.

◆ ❖ ◆

Kate
Texas, USA

My story begins in January of 2004. At some point in that dreary winter month, I began waking up with swollen hands. I was mildly perturbed, but pushed it to the back of my mind. I thought it must be from the dry heat, and made a mental note to drink more water.

One evening in February, I was walking the dog. It was a chilly night, about forty-five degrees. I wore gloves. I had noticed increasingly that I could not stand the cold anymore. I thought that because cold weather is infrequent in Texas, I was just not acclimated. When I returned home after about seven minutes outside, I noticed that a fingertip was white and numb.

"Honey, I have frostbite!" I exclaimed.

"Uh, you cannot get frostbite when it is forty-five degrees. That is not normal." This, from a husband who usually reminded me that I was a hypochondriac, now, he was telling me I am not normal. Uh-oh.

I quickly logged onto the Internet and typed in "fingers turn white in cold." I found lots of links about Raynaud's. Okay. Hmm. What about this weird swelling lately while I am at it? Keywords: Raynaud's and swollen hands.

Uh-oh. Link after link was about scleroderma. I called my primary care physician (PCP) and was seen the next day. An inflammatory panel showed a positive antinuclear antibody (ANA), with a homogeneous pattern. The nurse said it could be lupus, according to the pattern. Well, lupus is not fun. But I can live a 'near-normal' life span with lupus. I had already read about scleroderma. I did not want to go there.

Two weeks later I saw my first rheumatologist. He was dry and nearly completely devoid of personality. He sat behind a large wooden desk while he asked me a million yes-or-no questions off a clipboard. They took several X rays and tubes of blood.

During the two weeks between my appointments, I began to have flushing on my face and chest. On some days I felt like I was coming down with a cold or flu.

In the first week of March, I found myself behind the large wooden desk again. He asked how I had been, and then seemed not terribly interested. He interjected, "Well, the labs show you have the SCL-70 antibody, so that means you have scleroderma. And the ANA means you have lupus.

Your X rays show some thinning of the bones, so you will need a bone scan today."

He began writing prescriptions for me and dictating his report to my primary care physician while I wept. He pushed some pamphlets at me and sent me off to get a bone scan. I tried to ask questions about what this meant. Does this mean I am going to have the scleroderma all over, or just in one area? He only said, "If it is in your blood, then it is everywhere."

I was sobbing while waiting in line to pay, and finally a nurse pulled me into a room and answered some of my questions. She showed me that the doctor had written down "mild scleroderma", so it did not sound all that serious. However, I had already read about SCL-70, and I knew that it likely meant diffuse scleroderma and possibly a more serious course.

I saw a second rheumatologist the following week for a second opinion. I am not interested in seeing the first doctor ever again. You simply do not give someone such a serious and possibly grave diagnosis in that manner.

The new rheumatologist examined me and said he was one hundred percent certain I did not have scleroderma. He also said it was highly unlikely I had lupus. He reordered all the lab work and said he would be extremely surprised if it still showed SCL-70 antibodies. At this visit, my complaints were flushing, swelling in the hands that came and went, some wandering joint pain and stiffness, and mild fatigue. He recommended I see a dermatologist about my face. The dermatologist could not determine if it was rosacea or a malar rash. He took a biopsy from my back and sent it to the Mayo Clinic. Although they biopsied normal skin in order to test for systemic lupus, the biopsy came back positive for sub acute cutaneous lupus. It showed inflammation, to be sure. My rheumatologist has referred me to another dermatologist who specialized in these issues, to get a second opinion about the lupus diagnosis.

Meanwhile, the lab work came back still showing the SCL-70 antibody. So despite my rheumatologist's initial impressions of "no way," we may still be looking at an overlap syndrome.

So far, my complement levels, sedimentation rates, blood counts, urine tests and chest X rays are all still normal, and I am thankful for that. I have been having some acid reflux problems. I have been laying off the junk food and sweets and chocolate as a result, and I have finally dropped those last five pounds, which is also something to be thankful for: the scleroderma diet!

My family has reacted in various ways. My sister has told me she is in denial. She is just not letting herself "go there" yet. That is fine. I feel like I am a complete bore. Like the little old lady who complains about her bursitis! I think my husband gets tired of hearing me tell him about my symptoms. I am thankful for the online forums out there.

I have had some people try to blame this on diet or diet colas, or on personal beliefs. I think it scares people to be reminded that some issues of our health are completely beyond our control.

I have had many strange symptoms come and go. I do not know whether they are from lupus or from scleroderma, but I suppose it does not matter. I have had unusual sensations on my skin, like someone sprinkling cold water on me. Sometimes I will touch my arm and look up, wondering if it was a raindrop or if the roof is leaking. One morning I woke up with a numb toe, and one day with a numb patch of skin on my arm. Sometimes my thighs get red and irritated, and they hurt when I walk.

My tongue is really strange looking. It is very cracked in the front and splotchy in the back. My rheumatolgist just said, "Blech! Be sure to show that to the dermatologist!" The dentist just said, "Hmm...it does look weird. But as long as it does not hurt...."

I have also been having temporomandibular joint (TMJ) symptoms off and on, and pain and a nodule in my wrist. My ankles are very noisy, as is my neck; lots of crackling sounds. Everything with this disease or diseases seems to be off and on. One day it is this, another day it is that, another day it is everything.

The last few days, I have been feeling rather normal, I am happy to say. I have had normal energy levels and less swelling. I am trying to hold onto these days and keep them in my mind so I can remember when things go sour that they can get better. I am not looking forward to the changes that may be coming, but I am tired of worrying.

If scleroderma was a person, he would be the biggest jerk alive. He is not someone I want to associate with. He may make himself very hard to ignore, and he may beat me up a bit, but I am not going to let him get the best of me.

Let us all keep hope alive for a truly effective treatment and ultimately a cure for this hateful disease.

◆❖◆

Lisa Williams
Massachusetts, USA

Hi, my name is Lisa. I am thirty-nine years old and I have had sclero-derma for eleven years. I am Native American and black. I am married and have two children, ages sixteen and thirteen.

My mother also had this disease for over twenty-three years and died seven years ago from complications. I also have a first cousin diagnosed with this disease three or four years ago. I have lived most of my life in Boston, Massachusetts.

I can remember when I was a child, playing in the snow and my hands becoming so cold and numb, probably because of Raynaud's, that I had to literally put them on the furnace to warm them. So I think I have had early symptoms long before I knew it.

Before my mom was diagnosed the doctors told her it was all in her head and to get rid of her husband and kids because we were making her sick and crazy. I still remember the day she quit her job and was disabled. She looked okay because she had scleroderma with no skin involvement. They told her she had about one to two years to live, so every one of those extra twenty-three years were definitely a blessing!

I knew I had scleroderma, but it took over a year to diagnose me. Finally when my skin hardened the doctors had to agree.

The first five years were difficult because I was so tired and fatigued. My arms were bent and my skin was hardening. I looked like I had been in a fire. My fingers are slightly bent. I remember not being able to bend down and tie my daughter's shoes. That really bothered me.

I took several different medicines but doctors could not prove that the medicine would help and I did not want to be a guinea pig so I have not used medication for over eight years now. I also believe that all those medicines and painkillers are what killed my mom, and not the scleroderma!

For all of my eleven years with scleroderma I have had a great rheu-matologist, Dr. Robbins, from Harvard Vanguard in Boston, MA. He listens and really cares. He also has called to check on me because he says I wait too long to check in with him and that I downplay my disease experience and/or symptoms.

I am still pretty active. I wake up stiff and tight, but I still work full time. Do not get me wrong, I know that I am sick because I am always very tired and cranky, and my joints ache all over. But I have no more skin hardening and no internal damage yet. People are amazed when I tell them I have scleroderma as I look so normal. I no longer fear scleroderma, I challenge it.

On a sad note, I was recently diagnosed with multiple sclerosis (MS). That also took over a year to diagnose. My doctors tell me that I am one out of millions with this case of bad luck.

I am now very involved with my diseases and medicines.I use the internet often to research. I am worried and nervous. You feel like you finally have a grip on life then BAM! But I will be okay.

I would like to meet anyone else with scleroderma and MS. I raised two children while having scleroderma and I have lots of suggestions and stories. My children have even written papers for projects on scleroderma for class.

Silezia Pretorius
South Africa

I am twenty-nine years old. I have been diagnosed with CREST. It took along time for the doctors in South Africa to find out what was wrong with me.

I was twenty-three when the first symptom presented itself. I always had a tendency to feel cold, like my blood circulation was just bad. I was working late one night and my colleagues noticed that my hands went black. They asked if I worked with ink. Of course I did not and mentioned that I am very cold (and it was the middle of summer in Africa!).

My fiancé rushed me to my general practitioner that evening and he diagnosed me with Raynaud's. He referred me to a specialist surgeon, who tested me for lupus. He then referred me to a rheumatolgist. She confirmed that I had systemic lupus erythematosus (SLE). They basically referred me to the Internet if I needed to find out more. I was shocked when I read about all the symptoms. The doctors put me on cortizone and Iloprost for six days in the intensive care unit (ICU). It did not work!

About one and a half years after being diagnosed with SLE, I started to experience additional symptoms of difficulty swallowing and difficulty using my hands and joints. I went back to the rheumatolgist. She ordered a barium swallow and X rays. She confirmed a day later that I had CREST. Again she referred me to the Internet and said that she will prescribe pain killers if I need them.

I was terribly upset as it seemed that the doctors in South Africa have limited knowledge about the treatment of the disease and there are no support groups that I could find. I emailed a scleroderma organization in America for help. They sent me information about a doctor in South Africa, whose office is just a block away from where I work.

He examined me, and ordered blood work, X rays, lung functions and a gastroscopy. He immediately confirmed CREST, but also SLE as well as Sjögren's. I am now diagnosed with mixed connective tissue disease (MCTD), with scleroderma being the dominant one.

He changed my diet and gave me vitamin supplements. He convinced me to try some natural remedies to relieve the symptoms. After about two years of eating right and using homeopathic treatments, my skin condition has improved tremendously, my mobility has improved, and I rarely get joint and muscle pain. The only problem that we cannot seem to manage is the reflux, but I try to manage it with my diet. The reflux is particularly bad due to the hiatal hernia I also have.

I follow an exercise program twice a week for an hour. I stretch a lot and I do Kata boxing. I practice pilates and yoga. I stay clear of proteins such as meat and eggs. I also avoid take-aways and fast foods. I eat a lot of fresh raw vegetables, fruit and fiber.

I sleep rather poorly, but the exercising seems to help for the insomnia. I also take care of my skin by exfoliating twice a week, and applying a moisturizing mask. I use a lot of moisturizer. I brush my teeth three times a day and I visit the dentist every six months. I also take fluoride supplements.

I believe that if we try to feel positive about our life and the cards we are dealt, then we can manage our disease most effectively. It seems to me that the more negative we are, the sicker we get!

PART 4

International

CHAPTER 9

Español (Spanish)

Asociación Colombiana de Esclerodermia
by Francisco J. Castellanos
ISN Líder Del Grupo De Ayuda. Bogotá, Colombia.

Hacia el mes de Junio de 2004 y luego de constatar que no existe en todo el país una Entidad Estatal o Privada que reúna a las personas que padecen de Esclerodermia, nace la iniciativa de crear una Asociación que agrupe a estos pacientes y a sus familias en Colombia. Es así como nace la Asociación Colombiana de Esclerodermia (ASCLER).

Para fortuna de todos los afiliados de ASCLER desde el momento mismo de su fundación, la Asociación ha estado afiliada a la Red Internacional de Esclerodermia (International Scleroderma Network), y gracias a ello, ha contado con invaluable apoyo informativo y con importantes herramientas logísticas como por ejemplo el alojamiento de información en el prestigioso sitio en Internet sobre esclerodermia: www.sclero.org.

En un comienzo la Asociación realizó reuniones únicamente con personas con Esclerodermia y/o con sus familiares, entre quienes se intercambió información de acuerdo con la experiencia personal de cada una de ellas respecto de la enfermedad. Pero, pronto se hizo necesario que ASCLER extendiera un poco más sus objetivos y alcances, por ello se programó la primera conferencia dirigida por un especialista médico Reumatólogo. También se invitó a participar de nuestras reuniones a personal empleado en Laboratorios Farmacéuticos y a Estudiantes de Universidades con facultad de Medicina Dermatología y Reumatología dando así a conocer la Asociación entre la comunidad médico-científica.

De igual manera, se estableció el Programa Esclerodermia con Calidad de Vida en desarrollo del cual tanto los pacientes como sus familiares han obtenido grandes beneficios que les han permitido mejorar sus condiciones físicas y anímicas.

Buscando ayudar a la gran mayoría de pacientes en todo el territorio del país, la Asociación también ha elaborado diferentes folletos con información sobre la enfermedad, algunos de estos se denominan: Aspectos Generales de la Esclerodermia; Esclerodermia Sistémica Difusa; Esclerodermia Localizada; Síndrome de C.R.E.S.T. Estos folletos plegables contienen un compacto resumen acerca de cada tipo de esclerodermia y han sido revisados y corregidos por el Dr. Luis Catoggio, prestigioso Reumatólogo argentino, miembro de la Junta Consultiva Médica de La red Internacional de Esclerodermia -ISN Medical Advisory Board- y son enviados a todos los centros médicos del país, Clínicas y Hospitales, que cuentan con servicio de Reumatología y/o Dermatología para que sean los propios médicos especialistas quienes los entreguen a los pacientes cuando éstos acudan a la consulta médica.

La Asociación ha venido ganando adeptos, afiliados y colaboradores, teniendo un objetivo fundamental definido: El mejoramiento de la Calidad de Vida de los pacientes con Esclerodermia y sus familiares a través de un mejor conocimiento de la enfermedad, su tratamiento y los cuidados generales que estas personas deben observar y ofreciendo orientación, información, esperanza y ayuda a toda la comunidad afectada por Esclerodermia.

Cualquier persona que desee participar de estas actividades es bienvenida a ASCLER y podrá contactar directamente con nuestra sede ubicada en la Carrera 10 N° 20-19. Oficina 606-A de Bogotá D.C. o consultar sobre ellas a través de Internet en el sitio: www.sclero.org.

Rodolfo E. Claudet
Morfea
Peru

Este relato fue traducido del español al ingles por Edwin Lamoli-Torres, quien es un profesor retirado de la Universidad de Puerto Rico-Recinto de Mayaguez. La version en ingles de este relato esta en el capitulo 6.

Hola! Mi nombre es Rodolfo. Hace un anio fui diagnosticado de esclerodermia localizada (morfea).

Y recibi asistencia por una Dra aqui en Peru. Y por motivos que no puedo entender no pude seguir con el tratamiento. Tengo lesiones en la espalda y e notado que me estan saliendo otras junta a las que ya hay.

Espero tus consejos y sugerencias.

CHAPTER 10

Italiano (Italian)

Al
Sclerodermia con Sindrome di Raynaud
Italia

This story was translated from Italian to English by Kevin Howell. He is a Clinical Scientist for Professor Black at the Royal Free Hospital in London. The English version of this story is in Chapter 5.

Salve, ho 30 anni, maschio e dal 1998 mi sono iniziati problemi di circolazione agli arti superiori, soprattutto alle dita delle mani (indici), con perdita parziale o totale della sensibilità in particolari condizioni climatiche (freddo, oppure a conntatto con l'acqua di mare d'estate), con pallore e colorito bluastro.

Al momento non gli ho dato molto peso, poi col passare del tempo ho notato sulle punte delle dita delle incavatura che mi provocavano moltissimo dolore: all'inizio sembrava che crescessero delle specie di piccole unghiette o pellicine molto spesse verso l'interno delle dita. Con qualche piccola escoriazione o ferita notavo che ci metteva molto tempo a guarire perché la crosticina cresceva verso l'interno e non verso l'esterno.

Poi mi sono iniziati dolori alle braccia e gambe, dolori alle articolazioni (come l'artrite reumatoide), gonfiore alle mani, aumento di peso, ma fino a quel momento non presi nessun antidolorifico. Da due anni sono in cura presso il reparto seconda medica dell' Ospedale Maggiore di Trieste.

Ringrazio tutto lo staff medico che mi ha diagnosticato la sclerodermia; perché non c'è niente di peggio dell'ignoranza o il non sapere come e cosa affrontare; e di come portare a conoscenza dei familiari o degli amici.

◆ ❖ ◆

Alessandra Brustolon
Morphea
Italia

This story was translated from Italian to English by Kevin Howell. He is a Clinical Scientist for Professor Carol Black at the Royal Free Hospital in London. The English version of this story is in Chapter 6.

Alessandra, 40 anni, da circa un anno e mezzo mi è stata diagnosticata la Morphea. Ho macchie solo sul lato destro del corpo: coscia posteriore,fianco e zona inguinale.Le mie macchie sono rossastre-marroni e la pelle non è indurita. Ho iniziato con un forte prurito (specialmente sulla gamba) ma non ho mai avuto dolore. Ultimamente la macchia della zona inguinale si è allargata, nonostante i medici del San Lazzaro (TO) avessero visto al microscopio che la malattia fosse in fase regressiva.

Angela G.
Sindrome di Sjögren e il Lupus Eritematoso Sistemico
Italia

This story was translated from Italian to English by Kevin Howell. He is a Clinical Scientist for Professor Carol Black at the Royal Free Hospital in London. The English version of this story is in Chapter 8.

Sono Angela dalla provincia di Pesaro, ho 29 anni e da qualche tempo ho scoperto di avere la Sindrome di Sjögren e il lupus eritematoso sistemico. Sono anni che soffro per dolori alle ossa (specialmente mani, braccia e ginocchia) ma pensavo che il disturbo poteva essere provocato dal fatto che ero donatrice di sangue, per cui decisi di non donarlo più.

Quando mi sposai ebbi un figlio e con la gravidanza passarono tutti i dolori. Dopo 4 anni provai ad avere il secondo bambino che purtoppo persi a poche settimane. Da lì cominciai ad ammalarmi sempre con coliche addominali, cistiti, candidosi, congiuntiviti con corpi citoidi ovaliformi attaccati agli occhi, faringiti, abrasioni corneali, febbre, scarlattine, stomatiti, gengiviti e afte, sonnolenza-stanchezza, vertigini, paresi facciale e tornarono i dolori alle articolazioni. Ebbi un secondo aborto dopo del quale ricominciai a stare meglio.

Dopo altri 2 anni finalmente riuscii ad avere un secondo figlio. Mentre allattavo mi tornarono quei dolori alle articolazioni, ma pensavamo fossero causati dall'allattamento, quando smisi di allattare i dolori non cessarono.

Ai vari disturbi si associarono le vertigini finchè una domenica sera ho avuto per circa 2 ore vertigini acute, difficoltà respiratoria, oscuramento della vista, sudorazione, formicolio alle gambe e quando provavo a camminare tendevo ad andare verso sinistra. Abbiamo chiamato un'ambulanza e da lì sono cominciate tutte le visite ed esami (otorino, neurologo, reumatologo/risonanza magnetica, analisi del sangue, prove per quantificare la salivazione e lacrimazione, controllo della pressione nelle 24 ore , prove vestibolari, audimetriche etc.).

All'inizio si pensava fosse sclerosi, ma la risonanza l'ha esclusa. Il reumatologo ha sospettato subito la sindrome di Sjögren, mentre per riconoscere il lupus mi sono ricoverata per esami specifici nella clinica Reumatologica di Jesi. Così attraverso le analisi del sangue, visita reumatologica e ricovero, mi hanno diagnosticato queste due malattie.

Ora so che i miei dolori andavano e venivano con le gravidanze(queste malattie sono collegate in qualche modo con gli ormoni) e so anche che dovrei cercare di non avere altri figli. Non so ancora che percentuale di probalità hanno i miei figli nell'avere queste patologie. Inoltre nel lavoro che svolgo ho difficoltà di movimenti e di restare attiva(spesso sono stanca), vorrei sapere se chi ha questa malattia riesce a lavorare normalmente.

Anghelita
Sclerodermia di Zia Lia
Italia

This story was translated from Italian to English by Kevin Howell. He is a Clinical Scientist for Professor Carol Black at the Royal Free Hospital in London. The English version of this story is in Chapter 4.

Io sono la nipote di Zia Lia, che purtroppo non é più qui con noi, la sua malattia é stata dolorosissima e galoppante, dalla data della diagnosi ha vissuto solo tre mesi. Sono stati mesi di sofferenza per lei e per tutti noi e soprattutto per le suo figlie di 16 e 18 anni. Io la voglio ricordare per la sua allegria e gioia di vivere aveva 46 anni, era bella e con un sorriso che arrivava al cuore.

La su malattia inizialmente ha avuto il suo decorso con le ulcere alle dita delle mani, poi all'ispessimento e al pallore del viso, pian piano di tutto il corpo, poi è entrata dentro e le ha colpito i reni, da qui ha iniziato a fare dialisi, poi ha colpito il cuore e alla fine la sua morte é avvenuta per soffocamento.

Non dimenticherò mai quel viso sofferente e amorevole con tutti. Questo é avvenuto nel 1984 io ero una ragazzina. Il ricordo di Zia Lia è sempre vivo in me.

◆ ❖ ◆

Carlo Hernandez
Sclerodermia o Sclerosi Multipla
Venezuela

This story was translated from Italian to English by Kevin Howell. He is a Clinical Scientist for Professor Carol Black at the Royal Free Hospital in London. The English version of this story is in Chapter 7.

Nel 1997 o presso un forte rasfredore, a la settimana, caminavo e perdevo il equilibrio. Parlavo come se fosse ubriaco, dolori ne le gambe, le bracci la testa tutti i giorni. Doppo 4 settimane mi hanno referitto a una neurologo, mi ha fatto la evaluazione e mi aveva detto che avevo i sintomi del Sclerosi Multipla.

O ricevutto Solumedrol 1gr per 5 giorni e mi o ricoverato un 60%. Ne la RM non ció placche nel cerbello e ne anche la medula, o neuropatia ottica nel occhio sinistro e la elettromiografia avevo una picolla variazione nel occhio sinistro e nel orecchia sinistra. Io ero Pilota di una Linea Aerea cui in Venezuela. Sono anche italiano per mia mamma.

O perso il mio brevetto di volare per questo inconveniente. Oggi giorno a mia dottoressa e un po confussa perche mi dice che cio sintomi che non si relazionanno con la Sclerosis, per dire, sempre o i dolori e giá sono quasi 7 anni e mi diccce che per la mia condizione, e per avere placche nel cerbello.

Vorrei sapere se conscette del Cerebelar Thoracic Outlet Sindrome o Sindrome di Raynaud che si asomilia a la sclerosi.

◆ ❖ ◆

Cervetti Marzia
Morphea
Italia

Spero solo che ognuno riesca ad uscirne fuori senza troppi problemi.

Sono una ragazza di 19 anni. Due anni fa andai a farmi visitare per delle macchie, ma solo ora sono venuta a sapere di cosa si tratta. Mi hanno detto che sono affetta da morphea, ma non mi hanno voluto spiegare di che cosa si tratta.

Io per ora ho solo queste macchie, alcune piccole e sparse di varie forme irregolari sul polso e due classiche ovali vicino all'inguine. Quelle al polso non hanno mai avuto chiazze bianche, mentre le altre vennero fuori direttamente con le chiazze dure bianche all'interno color avorio.

Mi dettero una cura - non ricordo quale - e mi andarono via solo le chiazze chiare. All'epoca, però, non dissero cosa avevo. Così non tornai a farmi ricontrollare. Mi fecero una biopsia e mi dissero che era tutto a posto. Perciò non gli detti molto peso, finchè quest'anno non mi accorsi che le macchie al polso stavano aumentando. Allora sono tornata a farmi visitare e mi hanno parlato di questa morphea.

Tuttavia, non mi hanno spiegato cosa era, non me lo hanno voluto dire. Così ho iniziato ad informarmi da sola. Ora sto seguendo una terapia: 3 capsule di piascledine a pasto (9 capsule al giorno) e una pomata al cortisone (Elocon) ogni sera. Mi hanno detto di farlo per sei mesi (fino ad ottobre), ma per il momento non noto cambiamenti. Talvolta le macchie si schiariscono un po', ma poi ritornano (quelle al polso lo facevano anche prima).

Grazie a questo sito sto iniziando a capire un po' meglio la situazione. Mi piacerebbe scambiare informazioni con chi ha il mio stesso problema, anche se per ora io posso dire ben poco. Spero solo che ognuno riesca ad uscirne fuori senza troppi problemi. Un grosso augurio a tutti.

◆ ❖ ◆

Iris C
Morphea-Guarita e Sindrome di Reynaud
Italia

La morphea si è fermata definitivament.

La mia storia inizia quando avevo 3 anni e mia madre nota sulle gambe delle piccole macchioline, in corrispondenza di precedenti iniezioni di penicillina, va dal medico che minimizza. Passano 2 anni e queste macchie non spariscono.

Mia madre va dal dermatologo che diagnostica infaustamente la sclerodermia e che sentenzia non c'è nulla da fare. Alla disperazione di mia madre (cui comunque non era stata data alcuna spiegazione specifica in merito) assiste un giovane specializzando in dermatologia all' università di Verona che vuole visitarmi subito.

Iniziano così, grazie a questo medico, le cure che qui in Italia erano ancora sconosciute e le continue visite mediche e i ricoveri in ospedale.

Questo va avanti per cinque lunghi anni, nei quali, devo dire la verità, non ho patito dolore fisico di alcun tipo. La morphea si è fermata definitivamente, le uniche tracce della malattia si possono vedere solo sulle mie gambe, dove sono rimaste delle bruttissime cicatrici, ma non mi posso lamentare, sono guarita e questoè quello che conta.

Lancia
Amica di una Paziente Affetta da Morphea
Italia

Salve! Qualche giorno fa hanno diagnosticato ad una mia cara amica (27 anni) la sclerodermia: penso che la Morphea dalle descrizioni riportate nel sito. Tutto è partito dal fatto che aveva un dito della mano, sempre freddo e bianco.

Si è recata a Modena e qui è stata sottoposta ad un intervento, di cui non ricordo il nome tecnico, ma che praticamente consiste nello "sblocco" di vasi sanguigni.

In questa occasione le hanno diagnosticato la sclerodermia. Ora io mi chiedo: cosa c'entra l'intervento cui è stata sottoposta con la malattia diagnosticata?

Laura Schiavone
Sclerodermia Sistemica Diffusa
Italia

Sono una ragazza di 22 anni; all'età di 12 anni all'improvviso mi sono comparse delle macchie violacee sul ginocchio sinistro; all'inizio pensavamo ad un fungo di mare ma tempestivamente mia madre ha contattato un medico dell'ospedale Niguarda di Milano che dopo infiniti accertamenti mi ha diagnisticato la sclerodermia che nel mio casoè di tipo diffusa.

Ero così piccola quando mi hanno detto di avere una malattia di cui non avevo mai sentito parlare non potevo fare altro che continuare a giocare e vivere la mia vita come se tutto quello che mi stava succedendo non mi riguardasse.

La mia malattia ha sempre avuto un decorso molto lento tranne che per la macchie che comparivano a vista d'occhio ; La mia vita cominciava a cambiare giorno dopo giorno non potevo più correre veloce come prima non potevo piegarmi sulle ginocchia gli arti mi facevano male; Nel giro di un paio d'anni le macchie si sono allargate dal ginocchio sinistro per tutto il lato sinistro del mio corpo escudendo il torace; Quando le macchie ormai erano pronte a diffondersi anche sul seno ho avuto una grazia e la malattia come per incanto si è fermata!

Ormai sono cinque anni che faccio controlli periodici a Milano con- tinue analisi e fortunamente tranne il fattore estetico, i problemi di tipo gastro-intestinale e i muscoli che ogni tanto si fanno sentire, io sto bene. Sono felicemente sposata, solo pochi giorni prima del mio matrimonio mia madre mi ha detto che se la malattia non si fosse fermata io sarei morta dopo una lunga agonia, quando seppi questa cosa io mi arrabbiai perchè pensai al fatto che mia madre non era stata sincera con me ma adesso io le dico "grazie" perchè mi ha fatto vivere quegli anni che dovevano essere gli ultimi nel modo migliore, felice, "mi ha regalato la mia giovinezza," forse grazie a lei io adesso sto bene. Adesso vorrei un bambino ma ho molta paura di risvegliare la mia malattia ma grazie alla forza che questa malattia mi ha dato sono sicura che andrà tutto bene.

Io voglio dare un consiglio a tutti i miei fratelli e sorelle: non scorag- giatevi vivete una vita serena vivete ogni attimo perchè io sono sicura che la serenità mentale aiuta a stare meglio anche fisicamante. Grazie a voi che mi avete ascoltata, "grazie alla vita".

◆ ❖ ◆

Lele
Mia Madre e Sclerodermia
Italia

E' morta il 04.05.72 all'età di 48 anni.

La storia riguarda mia madre. E' morta il 04.05.72 all'età di 48 anni. Oggi ricorre il suo anniversario. Cominciò a stare male all'incirca l'anno precedente. Accusava spossatezza, dolori muscolari e da sempre soffriva di mal di testa. Fu ricoverata in ospedale nel mese di marzo del 1972 e curata per "artrosi".Nella fronte ad un certo momento le spuntarone delle macchie più scure rispetto alla pelle. Da lì forse i medici cominciarono a vederci più chiaro e dopo averle prelevato dei frammenti di pelle le fecero analizzare e, ironia della sorte il giorno della sua morte ci dettero l'infausta diagnosi. Non ho mai saputo che tipo di sclerodermia fosse.

Maria Rosa
Sclerodermia Sistemica Progressiva
Italia

Ho 43 anni e nel duemila mi hanno diagnosticato la sclerodermia sistemica progressiva dopo l'apparizione del fenomeno di Reynaud.

Ho iniziato nell'ottobre 2003 a Torino presso l'ospedale Mauriziano il trattamento con terapia infusionale di Endoprost principio attivo iloprost e ho notato subito miglioramento a livello di pelle più morbida devo dire che sono al primo stadio e mi si formano ogni 6 mesi dei piccoli ispessimenti su due polpastrelli delle dita delle mani ho un inziale interessamento a livello esofageo con ernia iatale e polmonare per cui sto facendo terapia cortisonica d'urto ma non so di avere questa malattia perchè sto benissimo. Ho sentito parlare di un nuovo farmaco il Bosentan, qualcuno me ne può parlare?

Monja Sanchini
Sclerodermia Cutane Morphea
Italia

Sono una ragazza di 25 anni, solare e piena di energia della città di Pesaro. Ho scoperto circa 5 mesi fa', tramite il dott. Arcangeli di Cesena,bravissimo ad aver riconosciuto da subito quello che potessi avere, di essere affetta da sclerodermia cutanea morphea.

Circa 1 anno fà, ho notato di avere dei duroni molto evidenti sulla pelle ed ero convinta che fossero delle cisti; infatti lo stesso dottore di famiglia mi diagnosticòche secondo lui non era niente di preoccupante e che nel caso si fossero ingrandite avrei dovuto sicuramente toglierle! Così tutto ebbe inizio,quando oltre ad aver colpito lo stomaco, queste, si presentavano anche sul dorso della schiena e lungo il braccio destro!

Mi venne detto dal chirurgo che non aveva mai visto una forma di questo genere e che sicuramente non erano cisti. Non mi sono fermata ad un solo parere, dopo avermi prescritto soltanto delle creme, e mi sono domandata...ma sarà questa la cura giusta? e ho continuato fino a quando un giorno mi si presentò l'occasione di potermi far vedere anche dal dott. Silvestrini facente parte dell'echip del dott..Di Bella.

Sono passate solo 2 settimane da quando ho iniziato la cura, vi garantisco che ero molto incredula in tutto quello che mi si presentava! Oggi mi sto rendendo conto che le macchie dure che ho si stanno lievemente ammorbidendo!non vorrei parlare troppo presto....ma sicuramenteèuna cura che non ha effetti collaterali come tanti medicinali che prendiamo; visto che lui è l'unico fino ad ora,ad avermi detto che bisogna intervenire da dentro, fermare questo meccanismo, che è tutta una forma di cellule non funzionanti, che impazziscono nel venire a contatto con un agente esterno!Io sono una serigrafia, lavoro con agenti e soluzioni chimici da circa 6 anni; sono convinta che ha in qualche modo hanno influito su di me!

Quale dottore può dire che non sia stato un agente chimico a farmi scatenare tutto questo? Il dermatologo dice che non è lui la causa; io mi chiedo perché visto che molti studi anche all'estero danno inf! ormazioni differenti! Oppure i nostri dottori non sono al avanguardia con il resto del mondo! Scusate sono tutte domande che ti poni quando ti trovi di fronte ad avere paura,che a soli 25 anni potresti iniziare ad aver problemi con i movimenti perché la malattia inizia a contrarti anche la muscolatura! Molti dottori dicono che la sclerodermia cutanea morphea non colpisca gli organi…ma siamo proprio sicuri di questo? Ho provato a fare domande su questo evitano di risponderti…loro ne sono sicuri, ma cure ancora non me ne hanno trovate!

Siamo un popolo ancora non capaci ad ascoltare chi può saperne più di noi,non diamo spazio a chi vuole tentare con delle cure diverse da farmaci tradizionali con più casi di diverso genere risolti, di provarci! Io sono ansiosa per la cura del dott. Di Bella.che sto facendo,ma se avesse ancora dei risultati…AMICI ve lo dico!

Sonia Spataro
Sclerodermia Sistemica Progressiva
Italia

Nel 1996 ho cominciato ad avere i primi sintomi di una malattia fino a quel momento sconosciuta a me e ai mei familiari.

Ho 39 anni e ormai da otto anni convivo con la sclerodermia. Tutto è iniziato con gonfiori diffusi agli arti, difficoltà di movimento, spossatezza e una diagnosi di Fenomendo di Raynaud in paziente autoimmune da seguire nel tempo.

Il tempo è stato breve perchè nel giro di pochi mesi la mia malattiaè esplosa. Attualmente oltre ai danni alle mani, perdita di sensibilità, ferite ulceranti e cattiva circolazione,- e macchie diffuse dal ginocchio in giù, ho problemi cardiachi (tachicardia parossistica sopraventricolare) che mantengo sotto controllo anche grazie a medicinali specifici quali dilatrend, enapren, aldactone. Sono andata in inghilterra al Royal Free Hospital di Londra dalla Prof. Carol Black che mi segue da lontano con l'aiuto di un bravissimo immunologo del II policlinico di Napoli. Mi hanno tolto il cortisone e mi hanno prescritto vitamine, olio di fegato di merluzzo, vit. A, C, D, E.

Insomma si lotta continuando a fare una vita più o meno normale, lavoro, marito, figlia, ginnastica ecc. Attualmente il problema più grosso è rappresentato dalle mani. Sono alla ricerca di qualcuno che mi possa indirizzare e indicare qualche struttura ospedaliera in grado di rendere le mie mani più "utilizzabili".

◆ ❖ ◆

CHAPTER 11

Nederlandse (Dutch)

Leon
Linear Scleroderma
The Netherlands

This story was translated into English by Ans Mens, and is in Chapter 6.

Bij mij ontdekte men op 5 jarige leeftijd twee vlekjes op mijn linker onderarm. Door de huisarts werd ik doorverwezen naar de dermatoloog, die kon er niets van maken en stuurde mij door naar de neuroloog. Hij moest ook wat onderzoekjes doen, waaronder de z.g. ruggeprik en een penicillinekuur per spuit.

Dit ben ik mijn gehele leven niet vergeten. Hij kon ook geen diagnose stellen. Dit speelde zich af in 1962 -1963. Dus werd ik door verwezen naar de dermatoloog in het Academisch Ziekenhuis te Leiden. Dit was in die tijd een wereldreis. Ik woonde toen in Zeeuws-Vlaanderen en het openbaarvervoer was toen helemaal niet goed geregeld. In het AZL weer een hele rits onderzoek, waaronder het wegnemen van een stukje huid/weefsel. Ik werd naar huis gestuurd met zalf, dat elke avond voor het slapen gaan op gedaan moest worden, mijn arm verpakt in plastic.

Dit heeft enkele jaren zo geduurd. In de tussentijd had men ook ontdekt, dat mijn linker pols niet kon buigen en mijn arm was minder ontwikkeld dan de andere. In het AZL werd ook doorverwezen naar een orthopedisch chirurg. Om mijn elfde werd ik geopereerd aan mijn arm, meer om te kijken hoe het er van binnen uitzag. Nu mijn spieren en pezen waren verbindweefseld.

In die tijd was ook de EMG ontdekt, dat heb ik dus ook mogen meemaken. Na mijn 12de jaar heb ik het ziekenhuis als patient niet meer van binnen gezien. De diagnose van mijn vlek wist ik nu ook, dermasclerose noemde men het toen. Maar er was niets aan te doen. Ik weet al jaren, dat ik een minder funktionerende linker arm/hand heb en daar heb ik mee leren leven. Op mijn 20ste zag ik het ziekenhuis weer van binnen, als.....verpleegkundige! Ik heb altijd goed kunnen funktioneren, ik wist en weet wat mijn beperkingen zijn.

Ik kreeg wel meer last van mijn pols, die ging steeds meer naar achter staan. Op mijn 25ste ben ik geopereerd door een orthopedisch chirurg aan mijn pols, hij heeft de pezen geprobeerd te verlengen d.m.v. klieven. In het vooronderzoek ben ik onderzocht door een hoogleraar dermatologie in het Academisch Ziekenhuis Nijmegen. Toen heb voor het eerst de definitieve diagnose vernomen, dermasclerose lineara en het is een kinderziekte, maar er is niets aan te doen. Maar ik weet nu iets.

De operatie heeft helaas niet het gewenste resultaat opgeleverd. Mijn beperking heb ik nog steeds. In de verpleging werk ik ook niet meer. Ik ben werkzaam als logistiekmedewerker. En nu op mijn 47ste wordt weer geconfronteerd men deze ziekte. Daar ik dagelijks achter de PC zit en veel de zelfde handelingen verricht heb ik sinds 1 1/2 jaar last van een pijnlijke linkerhand, vooral de vingers. Of ze met honderden naalden er in steken. RSI zei de huisarts en verwijst mij door naar de bedrijfsarts. Hem vertel ik mijn voorgeschiedenis en hij komt met een andere conclusie. Scleroderma is voor hem onbekend, maar hij zoekt het een en ander op. Leve het internet! Zijn diagnose is duidelijk, mijn scleroderma achtervolgt mij weer!

CHAPTER 12

Polski (Polish)

Maria
MCTD z Sclerodermia
Poland

W tej sytuacji tylko pozostaje mi wołanie o pomoc, bo życie bardzo szybko uchodzi,poprostu ta choroba zabija. Wielokrotnie hospitalizowana z rozpoznaną od 1997 roku mieszaną chorobą tkanki łącznej oraz szeregu współistniejących spraw chorobo wych, takich jak choroba Grawesa i Basedowa w w przebiegu choroby podstawowej, obecnie niedoczynność tarczycy, dolegliwości gastry czne,poważne zmiany posterydowe.

Bardzo są osłabione siły mięśniowe, głównie w zakresie kończyn dolnych. Ponadto obserwuje się znaczny obrzęk i zaczerwienienie twarzy z towarzy szącą dusznością, które mogą być wynikiem na tle alergicznym lub w wyniku choroby podsta wowej. Mimo wieloletniego postępowania klini cznego, ciągłej od wielu lat sterydoterapii oraz leczenia immunosupresyjnego stan mojego zdrowia pogarsza się.

W tej sytuacji tylko pozostaje mi wołanie o pomoc, bo życie bardzo szybko uchodzi,poprostu ta choroba zabija.

Conclusion
by Shelley L. Ensz

Voices of Scleroderma has shown us the height of courage of those who have lived, and died, with scleroderma and related illnesses. We have all given our stories—as patients, caregivers, survivors, and researchers—in the hopes of making it easier for others.

The three hundred stories in this series so far have just begun to tell the saga of scleroderma, which is so vastly different in every case with its onset, severity, symptoms, course and outcome.

Not even a thousand stories would clearly expose the dire and urgent need for more scleroderma information, support, awareness, and research throughout the world.

Yet, at the same time, every single story does tell the story of scleroderma; every single story does expose the need for a cure; every single story offers its own ray of hope, its own form of support.

Have you found solace and strength in this book and courage to continue your battle with illness or caregiving? Have you wept with grief or compassion from the stories of those who are suffering, or who have died?

Have their plainly detailed struggles whisked you away to seldom visited corners of your soul, changed the way you feel about your life, your health, your loved ones, your values, and the importance of cherishing each and every moment?

Whether or not you or a loved one has scleroderma or related illnesses, if you feel warmed by compassion and stirred to action by our plight of the "disease that turns people to stone," we invite you to continue to support the cause of scleroderma in your community and throughout the world.

By joining forces together, person by person and story by story, link by link, and group by group, someday our voices of scleroderma will be heard all around the world!

Someday, there will be a cure! And it will be because we all left our footprints on the sands of time.

"Let us then be up and doing, with a heart for any fate; Still achieving, still pursuing, learn to labor and to wait."

◆ ❖ ◆

Glossary of Medical Terms

A
acid reflux
A burning discomfort behind the lower part of the sternum usually related to spasm of the lower end of the esophagus or of the upper part of the stomach often in association with gastroesophageal reflux. *See also: heartburn*

alopecia
Hair loss or baldness.

amputation
Removal of part or all of a body part enclosed by skin.

antibody
A special protein produced by the body's immune system that recognizes and helps fight infectious agents and other foreign substances that invade the body.

antinuclear antibodies (ANA)
Antibodies or autoantibodies that react with components and especially DNA of cell nuclei and that tend to occur frequently in connective tissue diseases (as systemic lupus erythematosus, rheumatoid arthritis, and Sjögren's syndrome).

arthritis
Inflammation of a joint. When joints are inflamed they can develop stiffness, warmth, swelling, redness and pain. There are over one hundred types of arthritis.

aspiration pneumonia
Infection of the lungs due to aspiration (the sucking in of food particles or fluids into the lungs).

autoimmune disease
An illness that occurs when the body tissues are attacked by its own immune system, such as Hashimoto's thyroiditis, polymyositis, rheumatoid arthritis, scleroderma, Sjögren's syndrome, and systemic lupus erythematosus.

B
Barrett's esophagus
Metaplasia of the lower esophagus that is characterized by replacement of squamous epithelium with columnar epithelium, occurs especially as a result of chronic gastroesophageal reflux, and is associated with an increased risk for esophageal carcinoma.[1]

biopsy
The removal and examination of the tissue, cells, or fluids from the living body.[1]

bowel disease, inflammatory
A group of chronic intestinal diseases characterized by inflammation of the bowel, such as ulcerative colitis and Crohn's disease.

C

calcinosis

An abnormal deposit of calcium salts in body tissues, as is seen in some forms of disease, including CREST, which is a form of systemic scleroderma.

carpal tunnel syndrome (CTS)

A condition caused by compression of the median nerve in the carpal tunnel and characterized especially by weakness, pain, and disturbances of sensation in the hand and fingers.

CAT scan

A scan using computerized axial tomography.[1]

collagen

An insoluble fibrous protein of vertebrates that is the chief constituent of the fibrils of connective tissue (as in skin and tendons) and of the organic substance of bones.

connective tissue disease

Any of various diseases or abnormal stats (as rheumatoid arthritis, systemic lupus erythrmatosus, polyarteritis nodosa, rheumatic fever and dermatomyositis) characterized by inflammatory or degenerative changes in connective tissue.[1]

CREST Syndrome

A limited form of systemic scleroderma.

CT scan

A scan using computerized tomography.

D

diffuse scleroderma

A form of systemic scleroderma that generally involves widespread skin involvement.

dysphagia

Difficulty swallowing[1]

E

echocardiography

The use of ultrasound to examine and measure the structure and functioning of the heart and to diagnose abnormalities and disease.[1]

eosinophilic fasciitis (Shulman's syndrome)

A disease that leads to inflammation and thickening of the skin and a lining tissue under the skin, called fascia, that covers a surface of underlying tissues.

esophageal

Of, or relating to, the esophagus (throat).

esophagram

A series of X rays of the esophagus. The X ray pictures are taken after the patient drinks a solution that coats and outlines the walls of the esophagus. Also called a barium swallow.

ESR
Abbreviation for erythrocyte sedimentation rate.

F
fainting (syncope)
To lose consciousness because of a temporary decrease in the blood supply to the brain.
fibromyalgia
Any of the group of nonarticular rheumatic disorders characterized by pain, tenderness, and stiffness of muscles and associated connective tissue structures.

G
gangrene
Local death of soft tissues due to loss of blood supply.[1]
gastroesophageal reflux
Backward flow of the gastric contents into the esophagus resulting from improper functioning of the sphincter at the lower end of the esophagus.[1]
gastrointestinal (GI)
Of, relating to, or affecting both stomach and intestine.
GERD
Abbreviation for gastroesophageal reflux disease. A highly variable chronic condition that is characterized by periodic episodes of gastroesophageal reflux usually accompanied by heartburn and that may result in histopathological changes in the esophagus.

H
heart failure
A condition in which the heart is unable to pump blood at an adequate rate or in adequate volume.
heartburn
A burning discomfort behind the lower part of the sternum usually related to spasm of the lower end in association with gastroesophageal reflux.
hernia
A protrusion of an organ or part through connective tissue or through a wall of the cavity in which it is normally enclosed.
hiatal hernia
A hernia in which an anatomical part (as the stomach) protrudes through the esophageal hiatus of the diaphragm.
high blood pressure
Hypertension; abnormally high arterial blood pressure.
hypertension
Also known as high blood pressure; abnormally high arterial blood pressure.

hypothyroidism
> Deficient activity of the thyroid gland. A resultant bodily condition characterized by lowered metabolic rate and general loss of vigor.[1]

I
inflammation
> A local response to cellular injury that is marked by capillary dilatation, leukocytic infiltration, redness, heat, pain, swelling, and often loss of function and that serves as a mechanism initiating the elimination of noxious agents and of damaged tissue.[1]

interferon
> Any of a group of heat-stable soluble basic antiviral glycoproteins of low molecular weight that are produced usually by cells exposed to the action of a virus, sometimes to the action of another intracellular parasite (as bacterium), or experimentally to the action of some chemicals, and that include some used medically as antiviral or antineoplastic agents.[1]

interstitial cystitis (IC)
> A chronic idiopathic cystitis (bladder inflammation) characterized by painful inflammation of the subepithelial connective tissue and often accompanied by Hunner's ulcer.

irritable bowel syndrome (IBS)
> A chronic functional disorder of the colon that is characterized by the secretion and passage of large amounts of mucus, by constipation alternating with diarrhea, and by cramping abdominal pain.

J
juvenile scleroderma (JSD)
> Any form of scleroderma that afflicts children. The localized forms of scleroderma (such as linear and morphea) are most common in children.

K-L
limited scleroderma or **limited cutaneous systemic sclerosis (lcSSc)**
> A form of systemic scleroderma where the skin involvement is limited to the hands and/or face.

linear scleroderma
> A form of localized scleroderma, a line of thickened skin that can affect the bones and muscles underneath it, thus limiting the motion of the affected joints and muscles. It most often occurs in the arms, legs, or forehead, and may occur in more than one area. It is most likely to be on just one side of the body. Linear scleroderma generally onsets in childhood, and is sometimes characterized by the failure of one arm or leg to grow as rapidly as its counterpart.

localized scleroderma
> Scleroderma that affects only the skin and not the internal organs. Types of localized scleroderma include morphea and linear.

lupus

Any of several diseases (as lupus vulgaris or systemic lupus erythematosus) characterized by skin lesions. *See also: systemic lupus erythematosus (SLE)*

lymphoma

A usually malignant tumor of lymphoid tissue.[1]

M

migraine

A condition that is marked by recurrent usually unilateral severe headache often accompanied by nausea and vomiting and followed by sleep, that tends to occur in more than one member of a family, and that is of uncertain origin though attacks appear to be precipitated by dilatation of intracranial blood vessels.[1]

mixed connective tissue disease (MCTD)

A syndrome characterized by symptoms of various rheumatic diseases (as systemic lupus erythematosus, scleroderma and polymyositis) and by concentrations of antibodies to extractable nuclear antigens.

MRI

A procedure in which magnetic resonance imaging is used.[1]

morphea scleroderma

A form of localized scleroderma that affects only the skin, causing skin patches that may be red, brown, white or purplish in appearance.

multiple sclerosis (MS)

A demyelinating disease marked by patches of hardened tissue in the brain or the spinal cord and associated especially with partial or complete paralysis and jerking muscle tremor.

N

neuropathy

An abnormal and usually degenerative state of the nervous system or nerves; also a systemic condition (as muscular atrophy) that stems from a neuropathy.[1]

O

oesophagus

Alternate spelling for esophagus.

osteoarthritis

Arthritis of middle age characterized by degenerative and sometimes hypertrophic changes in the bone and cartilage of one or more joints and a progressive wearing down of apposing joint surfaces with consequent distortion of joint position usually without bony stiffening.[1]

P-Q

palpitations

A rapid pulsation; an abnormally rapid beating of the heart when excited by violent exertion, strong emotion or disease.

peripheral neuropathy
A problem with the functioning of the nerves outside the spinal cord. Symptoms may include numbness, weakness, burning pain (especially at night), and loss of reflexes.

petechiae
Pinpoint flat round red spots under the skin caused by intradermal hemorrhage (bleeding into the skin).

plaque, skin
A localized abnormal patch on a body part or surface and especially on the skin.

pleurisy
Painful and difficult respiration, cough and exudation of fluid or fibrinous material into the pleural cavity.

pneumonia
An infection that occurs when fluid and cells collect in the lungs.

prostaglandin
Any of various oxygenated unsaturated cyclic fatty acids of animals that have a variety of hormone-like actions (as in controlling blood pressure or smooth muscle contraction).

pulmonary fibrosis (PF)
Scarring throughout the lungs which can be caused by many conditions, such as sarcoidosis, hypersensitivity pneumonitis, asbestosis, and certain medications.

pulmonary function test (PFT)
A test designed to measure how well the lungs are working.

pulmonary hypertension (PH)
High blood pressure in the pulmonary arteries.

PUVA
PUVA stands for psoralen and ultraviolet A (UVA) therapy in which the patient is exposed first to psoralens (drugs containing chemicals that react with ultraviolet light to cause darkening of the skin) and then to UVA light.

R

Raynaud's or Raynaud's Phenomenon or Raynaud's Disease
A vascular disorder that is marked by recurrent spasm of the capillaries and especially of the fingers and toes upon exposure to cold, that is characterized by pallor, cyanosis, and a redness in succession usually accompanied by pain, and that in severe cases progresses to local gangrene.

reflux, esophageal
A condition wherein stomach contents regurgitate or back up (reflux) into the esophagus (throat).

rheumatoid arthritis (RA)
A usually chronic disease that is considered an autoimmune disease and is characterized by pain, stiffness, inflammation, swelling, and sometimes destruction of joints.

rheumatologist
A specialist in rheumatology, a medical science dealing with rheumatic diseases, which are any of various conditions characterized by inflammation or pain in muscles, joints, or fibrous tissue. Scleroderma is considered to be a rheumatic disease.

S

sclerodactyly
Scleroderma of the fingers and toes.[1] Swelling, tightening, curling, and hardening of the fingers and/or toes, as caused by the systemic forms of scleroderma.

scleroderma
A disease of the connective tissue. There are many different types of scleroderma. Some affect only the skin, while other types also affect the internal organs. *See also: diffuse scleroderma, linear scleroderma, localized scleroderma, morphea scleroderma,* and *systemic scleroderma.*

sedimentation rate
The speed at which red blood cells settle to the bottom of a column of citrated blood measured in millimeters deposited per hour and which is used especially in diagnosing the progress of various abnormal conditions.

seizure
Uncontrolled electrical activity in the brain, which may produce a physical convulsion, minor physical signs, thought disturbances, or a combination of symptoms.

Sjögren's syndrome
A chronic inflammatory autoimmune disease that affects especially older women, that is characterized by dryness of mucous membranes especially of the eyes and mouth and by infiltration of the affected tissues by lymphocytes, and that is often associated with rheumatoid arthritis.[1]

skin plaque
A plaque is a broad, raised area on the skin. Because it is raised, it can be felt.

stem cell transplantation
The use of stem cells as a treatment for cancer or other diseases.

systemic lupus erythematosus (SLE)
An inflammatory connective tissue disease of unknown cause that occurs chiefly in women and that is characterized especially by fever, skin rash, and arthritis, often by acute hemolytic anemia, by small hemorrhages in the skin and mucous membranes, by inflammation of the pericardium, and in serious cases by involvement of the kidneys and central nervous system.[1]

systemic sclerosis (SSc)
The type of scleroderma that can cause damage to skin, blood vessels, and internal organs. Subtypes include CREST, limited and diffuse scleroderma.

T

telangiectasia

An abnormal dilatation of capillary vessels and arterioles that often forms an angioma. (Plural: telangiectasias or telangiectases.)[1] Often casually referred to by patients as *red spots* or *red dots* on the face or hands.

thyroiditis, Hashimoto's

A chronic autoimmune thyroiditis that is characterized by thyroid enlargement, thyroid fibrosis, lymphatic infiltration of thyroid tissue, and the production of antibodies which attack the thyroid and that occurs much more often in women than men and increases in frequency of occurrence with age.

titer or **titre**

The strength of a solution or the concentration of a substance in solution as determined by titration.[1]

total parenteral nutrition (TPN)

Intravenous feeding that provides a patient with fluid and essential nutrients. Also referred to as *tubal feeding*.

tracheostomy

The surgical formation of an opening into the trachea through the neck especially to allow the passage of air.[1]

U

ultrasound

A noninvasive technique involving the formation of a two-dimensional image used for the examination and measurement of internal body structures and the detection of bodily abnormalities.[1]

undifferentiated connective tissue disease (UCTD)

When a person has symptoms of various connective tissue diseases without meeting the full criteria for any one of them, it is often called undifferentiated connective tissue disease.

V-Z

ventilator

Also known as respirator. A mechanical device for maintaining artificial respiration.

vitiligo

A skin disorder manifested by smooth white spots on various parts of the body.[1]

[1] By permission. From *Merriam-Webster's Medical Dictionary* © 2002 by Merriam-Webster, Incorporated.

◆ ❖ ◆

Index

Audrey Love Charitable Foundation xv
Australia 73, 110, 162, 167, 176, 185, 214
autoimmune 51, 67, 73, 96, 116, 272, 277, 278, 279
autoimmune hepatitis (AIH) 223
autologous stem cell transplant xiv, 7, 19, 155
Axelrod, Sari Hope 115
A Psalm of Life v

B
bacterial overgrowth syndrome (BOS) 12
barium swallow 79, 234
Barkett, Johnny 100
Barr, Amy 84
Barrett's esophagus 10, 33, 98, 272 *See also esophageal*
Bascom Palmer Eye Institute in Miami, Florida 115
Bast, Barbara "Bobbi" 126
bedridden 144
belching 12
Betancourt, Vanessa 178
Bethesda Naval Hospital 221
Betty 86
Beverly 87
biochemical abnormalities 26
biopsy 272
    deep tissue 195, 197
    skin 23, 73, 80, 82, 122, 171, 174, 182, 187, 221, 227, 230
        See also skin: biopsy
Bismarck, North Dakota, USA 141
Black, Professor Carol M. xv, 5, 124, 180, 207, 247, 248, 249, 251, 252
bleomycin 25
blisters 24
Block, Beverly Hutton 87
blood clot 39
blood pressure, high *See hypertension*
blood pressure, low *See hypotension*
blood pressure monitoring 17
blood thinners 115, 130, 142
blood transfusion 39
blueness (cyanosis) 8

About the Editors

Judith Thompson Devlin is Chair of the ISN Archive Development Committee and author of three published novels: *The Kiss of Judas*, *A Switch In Time* and *Mind Blindness*. She also collaborates with Shelley Ensz for the ISN's *Voices of Scleroderma* book series.

She resides in New Hampshire. She was diagnosed with CREST/systemic sclerosis in 1991 and has been on disability since then. Judith attended Dean Junior College in Franklin, Massachusetts. She holds a certificate for successful Hospice Volunteer Training and for Mediation Training.

She participated in a drug research program for scleroderma at the Boston University Medical Center with Dr. Joseph Korn as well as participated in the Scleroderma Family Registry and DNA Repository with NIH, presided over by Dr. Maureen D. Mayes.

Shelley L. Ensz is Founder and President of the nonprofit International Scleroderma Network, the Scleroderma from A to Z website, the Scleroderma Webmaster's Association, and EdinaWebDesign.com. She lives in Minnesota with her marvelous husband Gene, and their delightful Senegal parrot, Webstergirl.

The **International Scleroderma Network (ISN)** is a nonprofit organization that provides scleroderma medical and support information and works to raise awareness of scleroderma throughout the world. We also support international medical research for scleroderma through the ISN/SCTC Research Fund.

The ISN is an outgrowth of the Scleroderma from A to Z website at www.sclero.org, where the personal stories in this book were first published. Our website offers over twelve hundred pages of scleroderma medical and support information in twenty-two languages.

Over five dozen virtual volunteers from around the world operate the ISN website, book series, online support community, medical advisory, translation services, hotline, email support, and newsletter production services. We invite you to become an ISN member, donor and/or volunteer today, and help us tackle scleroderma!

Scleroderma Resources

International Scleroderma Network (ISN)
The ISN is a nonprofit, charitable organization that offers worldwide medical, support, and awareness information for scleroderma and related illnesses. See **www.sclero.org**.

EULAR Scleroderma Trials and Research Group (EUSTAR)
EUSTAR Scleroderma Centers are primarily in European countries. They diagnose and treat scleroderma patients as well as conduct research studies. See **www.eustar.org**.

Scleroderma Clinical Trials Consortium (SCTC)
The SCTC is a charitable, nonprofit organization dedicated to finding better treatment for scleroderma. Over 50 SCTC member institutions worldwide conduct clinical treatment trials for scleroderma, and they publish the Scleroderma Care and Research Journal. See **www.sctc-online.org**.

ISN/SCTC Research Fund
You may support international scleroderma research via the collaborative ISN/SCTC Research Fund, for top notch peer-reviewed international scleroderma research.

ISN's Scleroderma Webmaster's Association (SWA)
The SWA features Worldwide Support Group listings and the ever-popular *Scleroderma Sites to Surf!* Get your group or website listed today!

ISN's Scleroderma from A to Z Web Site "Sclero.Org"
The ISN operates Scleroderma from A to Z, where the personal stories in this book were first published. The website offers over one thousand pages of top quality scleroderma medical and support information in many languages. See **www.sclero.org**.

◆ ❖ ◆

ISN Membership and Donation Form

The ISN is a registered 501(c)(3) nonprofit agency based in the USA.
We send acknowledgements for all contributions.

❏ ISN Comprehensive Fund, Tackles Scleroderma on all fronts! Enclosed is my gift to ISN in the amount of $_____ (U.S. funds) to provide a powerhouse of scleroderma research, support, education and awareness.
❏ ISN/SCTC Research Only Fund. Enclosed is my gift in the amount of $_____ for international peer-reviewed scleroderma research.
❏ My donation is in loving memory of: _____

ISN Membership
❏ Email Membership. Enclosed is $25.00 or more (U.S. funds only) for an annual ISN Email Membership or Renewal (in English) to receive the ISN Insider Newsletter only by email.
❏ Postal Mail Membership. Enclosed is $35.00 or more (U.S. funds) for an annual ISN Postal Mail Membership or Renewal (in English) to receive the ISN Insider Newsletter through postal mail.

ISN Voices of Scleroderma Books:
❏ Volume 1: Enclosed is $25 per book (includes shipping) for _____ books.
❏ Volume 2: Enclosed is $25 per book (includes shipping) for _____ books.
❏ Volume 3: Enclosed is $25 per book (includes shipping) for _____ books

Notes:

Your Name (first, last): _____
Address: _____
City: _____ State:_____ ZIP:_____
Country: _____ Phone:_____
Email: _____

Pay by: Total: $_____ (U.S. funds)
❏ Check   Cardholder: _____
❏ Visa   Card #: _____
❏ Mastercard   Card Expiration Date: (month/year): _____
❏ AMEX   Verification Number: On the back side of your card, there is a long number. What are the last four digits? _____

Please mail this form with payment made out to:
International Scleroderma Network
7455 France Ave So #266
Edina, MN 55435 USA

◆❖◆

6428865R0

Made in the USA
Lexington, KY
19 August 2010